How to Give Yourself A Chakra Selfie

A Guide to Healing and Awakening Your Energy Body

SHERILYN BRIDGET AVALON

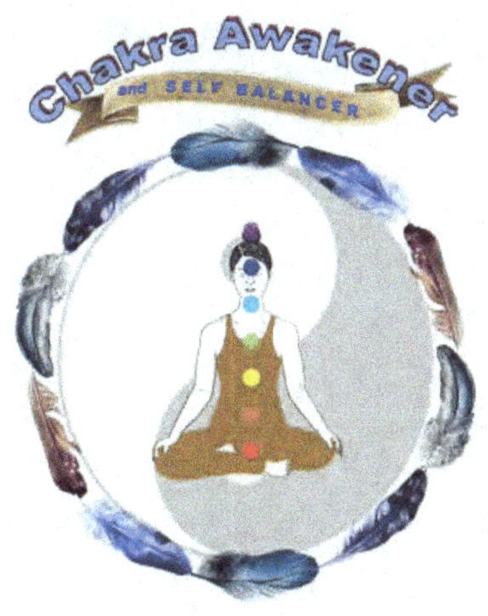

We are here to help you better understand our chakras, energy centers that govern different aspects of our body and mind. Chakras develops over our lifespan and can be related back to our physical, emotional and spiritual health. Awareness of each chakra can help us address old wounds and balance certain aspects of our lives. Issues such as scarcity mindset, lack of confidence, difficulty with expression, or trouble making decisions can be improved with this knowledge.

Our experiences and our ability to process emotions can affect our chakras development and when any one of them are imbalanced it will eventually affect the other chakras. When you bring your chakras to their original vibration, you can create more harmony within yourself and the world around you.

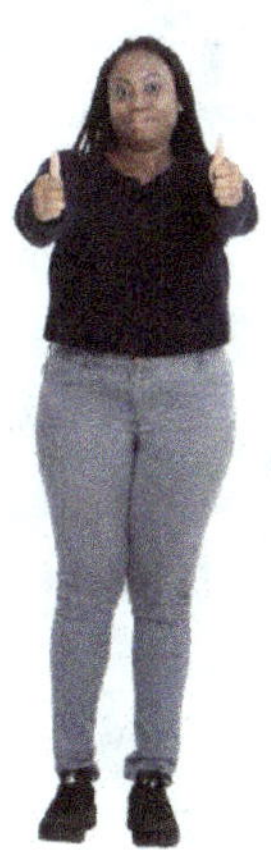

Table of Contents

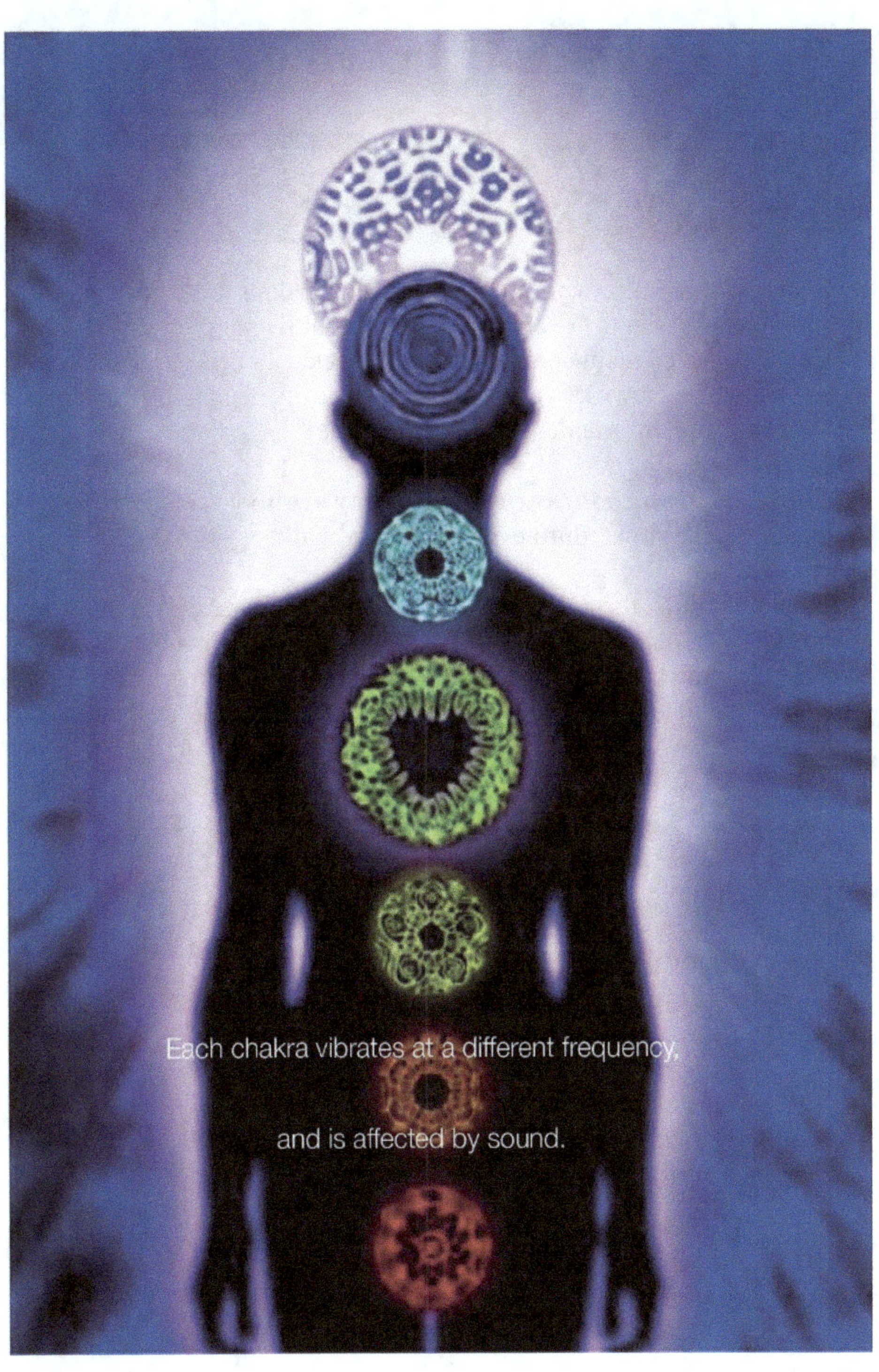
Each chakra vibrates at a different frequency,

and is affected by sound.

What Are Chakras Anyway?

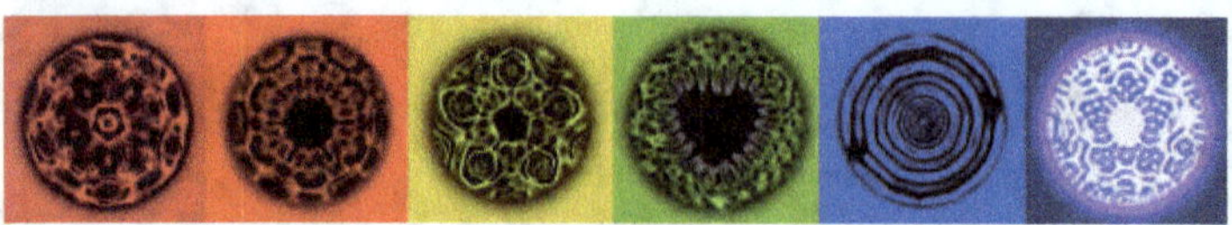

Chakra is a Sanskrit word meaning wheel. Chakras are wheels of energy, their centers are energy vortexes, that live in the subtle body. You have seven main chakras that are detected along your spine from its base to the crown of your head. These ideally need to be in balance for a happy, comfortable, and rewarding life.

The seven main chakras within the body are root, sacral, solar plexus, heart, throat, third eye, and crown chakra. (See page 19)

Throughout life, the balance of your chakras shift and move, they also go in and out of balance; the main reason is negative thinking. Awakening and balancing the chakras will help bring balance, harmony, and clarity into your life while releasing negative, stuck energy that no longer serves you or prevents you from reaching your highest potential.

Chakra balancing benefits

Experience the magic as you heal from within.

1. Overall, better health and well being
2. feeling energized and revitalized
3. increase in awareness of your higher self-connection.

The ultimate question is, do these feelings ever limit your ability to do something you enjoy? Answer is, yes! Imbalance, blockage, or disturbances in your energy centers or Chakras can create dis-ease and even ultimately result in physical illness.

By the thoughts we habitually entertain and act upon, we create the circumstances in which our life unfolds.
Paramahansa Yogananda

Chakra Awakening & Balancing Guide

The future of healthcare, simple techniques to

achieve whole body wellness in in just 7 days, you will discover all

you need to know to unblock and balance each of your 7 Chakras.

Session healing work performed is not a substitute for medical or psychological diagnosis and treatment. Intuitive healing processes offered are gradual, cooperative processes intended to enhance the clarity and expression of spirituality.

We know everything is energy & energy is frequency.

Einstein

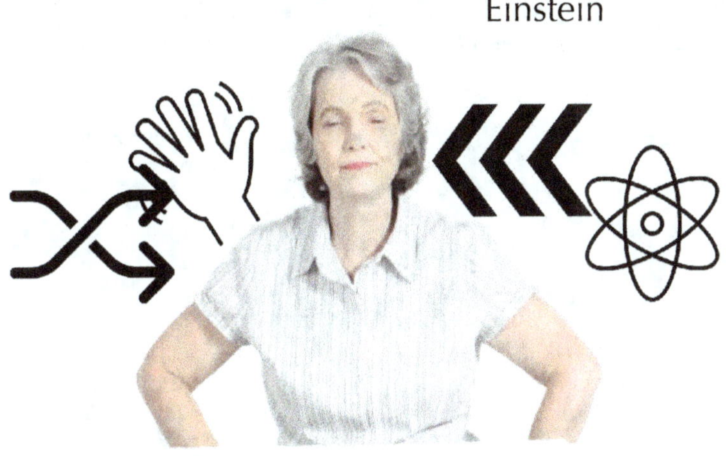

Frequency is the number of waves that pass a point in space during

any time interval, usually one second. We measure it in units of

cycles (waves) per second, or hertz. The frequency of visible light

refers to a color, and ranges from 430 trillion hertz, seen as red, to

750 trillion hertz, seen as violet. I like to use the acronym, **L.I.F.E.**

Living In Frequency Earth. Since this is where we are living.

How to Give Yourself A Chakra Selfie

It always helps if you learn the names, locations, and purpose of the energy of each Chakra.

A mantra is the speaking of a protected or secret word.

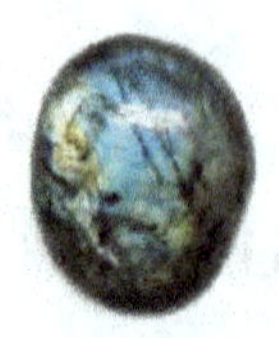

The Seven Chakras

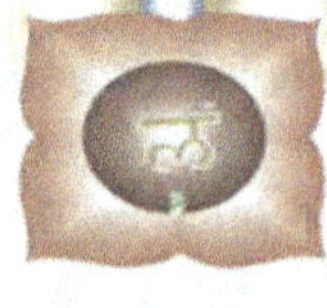

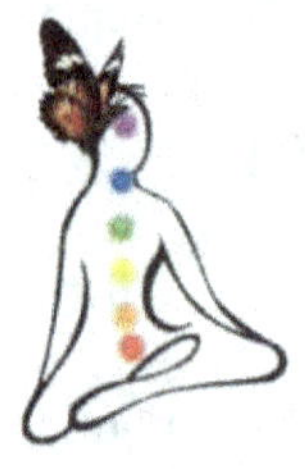

L.I.F.E
L i v i n g In
Frequency
Earth

"Bringing healing energy to the Soul of the world."

Your Chakras are the energy centers of your body, mind, and spirit. You can't see electricity and chances are you can't see your Chakras, but we know the power of electricity even though we can't see it and we don't understand it. We don't always understand our power system. In this course, we will walk you through **3 sets of Chakra Healing Exercises to help reprogram your system.** It's always better when you have a map, right?

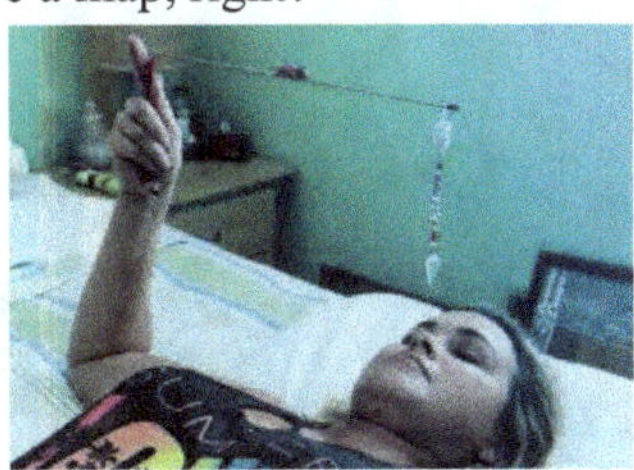

Chakra healing and clearing is maintenance; it is like changing the oil in your car, washing the sheets off your bed. If you don't look after your vehicle, what takes place? It breaks down. When those warm sheets come out of the dryer, what do you feel? The softness and warmth of a good night's sleep. We end up tired, depressed, obese, angry, and lost when we don't maintain our body's maintenance. When you regularly clean your Chakras, **you start to reverse decades of abuse** and fine-tuning of your body, so it is a **Ferrari instead of a 1960 Pinto**, that hasn't had an oil change in 6 decades.

The exercises take 5-30 minutes, and almost immediately, you will feel the blocked energies start to move out of your body. As you grow in knowledge and expertise through daily practice, you will tune in to your body and start knowing which clearing and healing exercises you need right now. As you tune your body it creates an entrainment field that helps you ascend to the next level of evolution.

The Seven Chakras

- The Chakra consists of seven levels that correspond to various systems of the body.

- The chakras are in the energetic body as opposed to the physical body.

- There are seven main chakras in your body, and they are shaped like a flower or a wheel, with petals or spokes that detail their composition.

- The chakras contain and process energy in your body, and just as energy can propel you, it can also block you.

- The chakras are like spinning balls of energy within your body like a series of cogs or wheels running up and down your spine working to continuously renew your energy.

- In a well-balanced, healthy person, the chakras move and spin rapidly and smoothly, and their colors are clear and bright.

- When you are stressed, ill or mentally impaired, your chakras get stuck, and they begin to slow down or even spin too quickly.

- They can even get discolored or fragmented if you are mentally, emotionally or physically impaired.

- Symbiotic with the Life force.

7. *Crown* - Cosmic **Physical Symptoms:** *Poor sleep habits, Cosmic Energy is not Flowing.* **When Blocked-** *Ego is in control, you feel lonely, depressed.* **Emotional Symptoms:** *feel a bodily disconnect with Spirit.*

6. *Third Eye* - Insightful **Physical Symptoms:** *Headaches, Hormonal imbalance.* **When Blocked** - *Illusion, depression, headaches. poor intuition.* **Emotional Symptoms**: *Poor intuition, Depression.*

5. *Throat* - Truth - **Physical Symptoms**: *Thyroid problem, Sore throat.* **When Blocked** - *lies, sluggish metabolism, thyroid problems, lack of expression, not following your truth.* **Emotional Symptoms:** *Can't express feelings, Heart and mind are disconnected.*

4. *Heart* - Love — **Physical Symptoms:** *Heart disease, High blood pressure.* **When Blocked** - *Grief, lack of Self Love, Self-pity, guilt, lack empathy, Lack forgiveness. Built a wall around your heart.* **Emotional Symptoms:** *Lack of empathy, Fear of intimacy.*

3. Solar Plexus - Will Power. - **Physical Symptoms:** *Poor digestion, Low blood sugar* **When Blocked** - *Shame, overblown ego, appetite, negative thinking, anger* **Emotional Symptoms:** *Low self-esteem, Lack of willpower, you get the feeling of butterflies, gut felt feelings, Silver cord is attached here.*

2. *Sacral* - Pleasure - **Physical Symptoms**: *Painful period, Infertility.* **When Blocked** - *Guilt, feel Self rejection,* **Emotional Symptoms**: *Low sex drive, creative block, low self-esteem, jealousy, blame, resentment, materialism.*

1. *Base/root* - Survival - **Physical Symptoms:** *Constipation, Fatigue,* **When Blocked** - *Fear, experience self-centeredness, greed, violence,* **Emotional Symptoms**: *Spacey, feeling unsafe, anxiety, fear. This is the foundation of which we build our life upon.*

How to Give Yourself a Chakra Selfie

Is color a manifestation of frequency?

We now have evidence of our Divine nature that we can physically feel. We know that specific frequencies are associated with specific chakras because we can physically feel each chakra when it is awakened by its corresponding frequency.

Keep in mind - the frequency generates the color. Color and frequency is the same thing perceived by different senses, which becomes relative to our perception.

Color is defined by the eye, and only indirectly from physical properties like wavelength and frequency. Since this interaction happens in a medium of fixed index of refraction (the vitreous humor of your eye) the frequency/ wavelength relation inside your eye is fixed.

We have both Male and Female spiritual energy, we call Feminale.

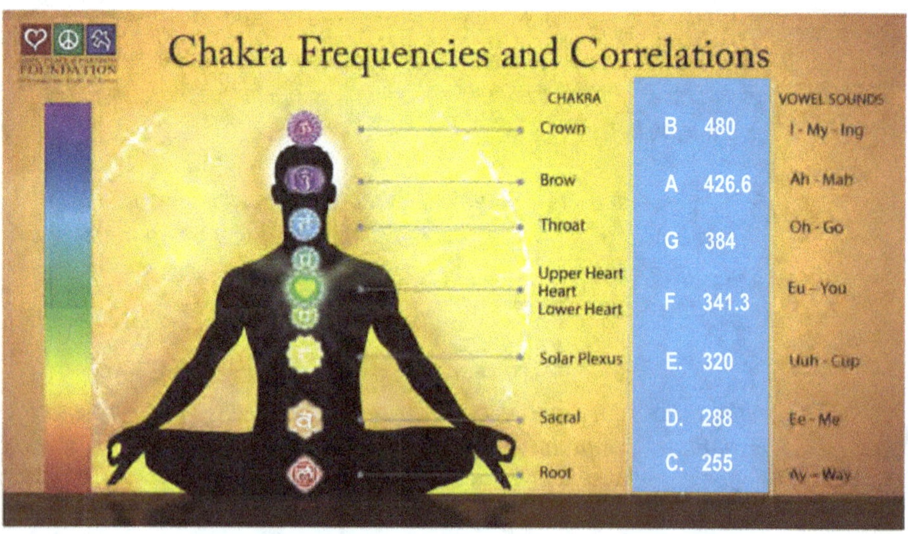

Giver from the Love, Peace & Freedom Foundation

"Why are Chakra Frequencies Important?"

You can't master that which you don't understand.

We, as empowered individuals, benefit by understanding our chakra system. For within this system lies the essential aspect of who we are as human spiritual beings.

Why are Chakra Frequencies Important?

- They provide us with tangible evidence that energy exists.
- They represent the reality of our innermost thoughts.
- Re-programming the Chakras are the key.
- We animate our physical body via thought frequency.

Ultimately, we are musical beings. Our challenge in life is to master our <u>Instrumental Self.</u>

The relationship between light, color, frequency, crystals, sound, chakras, and consciousness is part of the natural sciences. Necessary information every man, woman, and child should be made aware. If we are going to exist together as a community with integrity, our teachings must align with the reality of who we are as human spiritual beings.

Chakra Healing Modalities:

Healing is the voltage. The chakras activate energetic pathways into <u>nerve ganglia</u> and <u>organ systems</u> within the body. Then Energetic treatments can be constructed to a specific person's needs, using <u>music, intention, and the healing power from the human voice.</u> Within the treatment, we can combine a variety of frequencies that might include the vibrational rate through colored lights, energetics, or Chakra Selfie Healing, which will encourage and improve the body's natural healing abilities. ***In a nutshell color is frequency.*** The Quantum field is an invisible field of frequency this is where the Chakra Awakener creates a biological upgrade, by placing your attention on each Chakra.

Match the Chakra Symptom

Clearing your Chakras for better energy, better thinking. You must clear out the garbage clogging up your Chakra energy systems quickly and easily. **Remove the Cah energy that is built up by negative fear-based thoughts, or you will be full of Cah Cah.**

You may be the recipient of blocked Chakras if you experience:

A. Self-centeredness, greed or violence.
B. Feel self-rejection, low self-esteem, jealousy, blame, resentment or materialism.
C. Have an overblown ego or appetite, experience negative thinking, anger, talking too much.
D. Have lack of Self Love, experience guilt, self-pity, or instability.
E. Have a sluggish metabolism or weak will power. Inability to express yourself.
F. Have eye problems, headaches, bad dreams, or lack of concentration.

Match the

Chakra to the

symptom.

1. Throat

2. Crown

3. Root

4. Solar Plexus

5. Heart

6 Third eye

Answers:

1E, 2C, 3A,

4B, 5D, 6F

Meditate

Meditation is an absolute priority to begin opening and using your *Third Eye Chakra and the Pineal Gland.* While meditation may call to mind sitting in a lotus position and staring at a wall, it does not always need to look this way.

The point of reflection is to reach the alpha-state of your brain. The state where your mind is working at an optimum level. You can achieve this state in many ways, including showering, walking in nature, self-hypnosis, and even driving familiar stress-free roads. The key is to find what works for you to enter a deep meditative state and do it daily.

You are not likely to see immediate benefits from meditation. In some cases, it can take weeks or months to reap the rewards, especially if your chakras have been blocked for some time. Using the Chakra Selfie Stick is the best way to open your chakras quickly.

Find your Balance

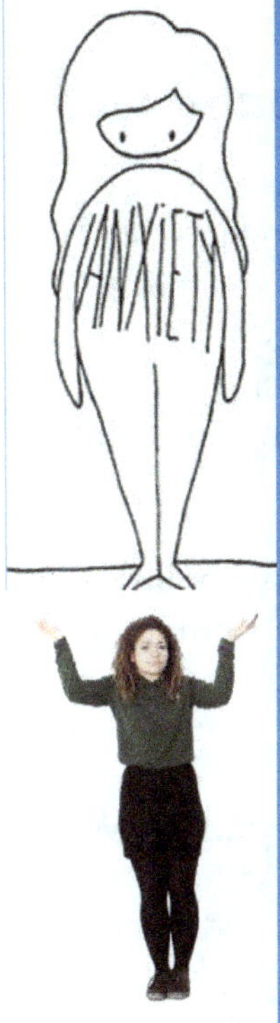

with Chakra Energy Healing

Exercise #1 Visualizing your chakras-

When you show more love, more abundance, more awareness, that's what you get as we affirm our self- worth and our choices for health, wealth, and ease of life our world changes. Let's analyze your routine thoughts. We need to simply attune to your specific needs and take time to invest in you.

By moving stagnant energy through your energy centers or Chakras, you may experience a reduction, or a release of negative emotions that often affect you daily life. During this process, some people experience the ability to set free old feelings, old thoughts, while freeing up new and clean energy to travel through their bodies.

Negativity and self-limiting thoughts block your energy. Once you begin the inner work of affirming your being and honoring who you are. Then deciding to start balancing your Chakras, your destiny will begin to unfold. Your life starts to change.

If we feel a particular way about something, will it affect the way we respond emotionally or, energetically to it?

Yes, remember energy is Consciousness.

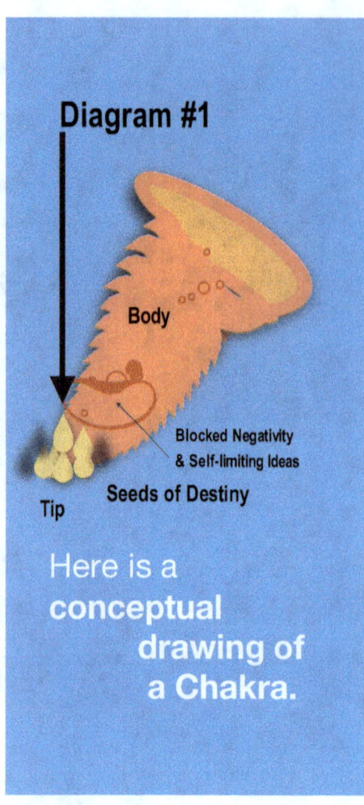

The universe responds to

what we think about ourselves.

A Chakra is divided into three sections: the outer lip, the body, and the tip. The outer lip of the Chakra acts as a filter to our daily exchanges with our surroundings. If our feelings remain unexpressed, this energy accumulates and congests in our energy system.

Blocked Chakras are causing symptoms of fatigue, aging, and illness. The main body of the Chakras comprises a delicate web of etheric energy.

We are composed of the warp and weave of our thoughts and attitudes. At the very core (or tip) of the Chakra are seeds. These seeds are of your destiny. The seeds cannot be opened until our negativity, and self-limiting ideas have been removed.

If energy follows thought…

As you open yourself to what is good and positive your destiny unfolds. Health, joy, prosperity, and wellbeing will emerge out of the "Seeds of Destiny" from the knowing that we deserve the life we say we want. We direct our destiny by managing the ways we think. We either become inner-directed or outer-directed.

Inner-directed is knowing our self-worth and goodness and experiencing ourselves as enough.

Outer-directed is dictated by family pressure, social and religious standards, and experiencing ourselves as not enough. If so, we need to create a pattern interruption and do a biological reprint.

How does Energy Healing work? Doing pattern interruption and a biological reprint.

Negative energies (thinking negative) are always around us. They are affecting your aura without you even knowing. Your aura is the principal source of catching negative energies. When negative energies are around you, they drain your positive power and make you feel sad and depressed.

The delicate balance of **aligning your chakras, grounding techniques, and consciousness re-patterning** affecting your aura will expand your consciousness to greater heights in a brief period. The old programs you once held as truth will melt away. **(Learn at your own pace. With the exciting holistic approach to understanding your energy system.)**

As I mentioned, our Chakras are the energy centers of our body. If all are not absorbing energy, not open, and not cleared periodically, it will lead to things like illness, depression, pain, relationship issues, and more. It's like changing the oil in your car regularly to keep it running smoothly.

Here's How Energy Healing works.

To start, you adjust your thinking, taking responsibility for everything you do and speak. Aligning your direction of thinking back to positive, which will then balance your energetic system to create a beautiful new you. We will show you how to change your life from the inside out. Too much exposure to negative energy affects your mental level and makes you feeble, and ill when depleted. When you regularly detox your body, chakras, and exercise, you reverse decades of abuse and begin fine-tuning your body.

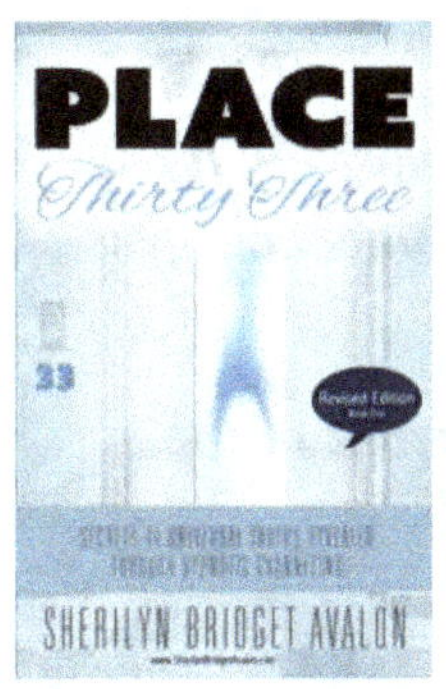

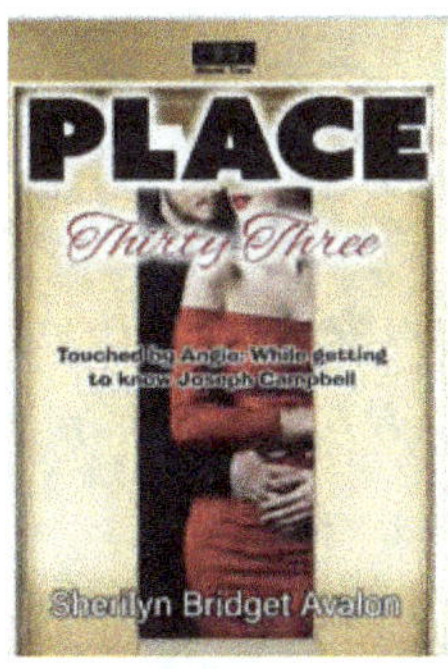

Get your copy of "Place 33, Secrets of Universal Truths Revealed" and "PLACE 33, TOUCHED BY ANGIE while getting to know Joseph. www.ascensions.us On our website. www.SherilynBridgetAvalon.com, or Amazon, or Barnes and Noble Today!

Most of these pathways are sealed in most people. They open through the intention to align while expanding their consciousness, or through spiritual purification work.

Since the Chakras serve to vitalize the physical body, they are directly related to the body's pathology or energy blockages.

Everything has its own aura, and often we can sense the auric field of a person when we pick up on their 'vibe', for instance, standing in line at the store.

The Chakras Major Functions:

It's good to connect to God/Source Every day.

1. **To vitalize the auric bodies and the physical body, organs, and glands.**

2. To bring about the development of different aspects of self-consciousness.

3. **Each Chakra is related to a specific, psychological, or higher mental blueprint, form, and function.**

4. To transmit energy between the auric layers of the Light-body. (Illustration C, pg. 21) Each auric layer of the body has its own set of seven major particle-wave Chakras, and eight corresponding anti-particle wave Chakras.

5. (Illustration C, pg. 18 *(also called morphogenetic chakras)* **each located in the same place on the physical body. Each successive layer exists in an increasingly higher Frequency, each with a higher frequency band more elevated than the lower one. *Energy is transmitted from one layer to the next through pathways in the tips of the Chakra.***

The daily practice of positive thought and chakra balancing Make an imprint into the Aether.

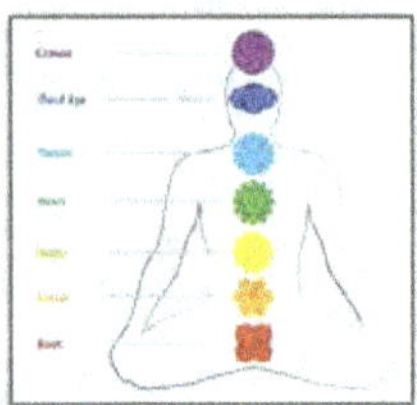

INTRODUCING THE CHAKRA AWAKENER

Chakra Awakener/ Selfie Stick

The Chakra Awakener emanates powerful positive vibrations while it speeds up the power of synchronicity in the user's life, bringing faith and action to the user.

1. The *Chakra Awakener* is also an abundance helper, attracting new positive relationships.
2. The *Chakra Awakener* stirs up creativity in the user.
3. The *Chakra Awakener* enhances and balances all energy centers.
4. The *Chakra Awakener* helps diagnose an imbalance in individual chakras.
5. The *Chakra Awakener* helps restore visualization, in Pineal Gland with deep breathing, which relaxes the mind.
6. The *Chakra Awakener* is also used to help in the **prevention of your dis-ease.** (before the thought of dis-ease arises.) See the explanation of *dis-ease.
7. The *Chakra Awakener* also provides safe exploration into another level of consciousness while facilitating a visionary experience.
8. The *Chakra Awakener* assists in revealing inner truths, intuition, and clarity.
9. The *Chakra Awakener* may also ward off psychic invasions, healing all auric holes.

Dis-ease - when Chakras are out of balance with the endocrine system, from your negative thoughts, emotions, and electromagnetic pollution.

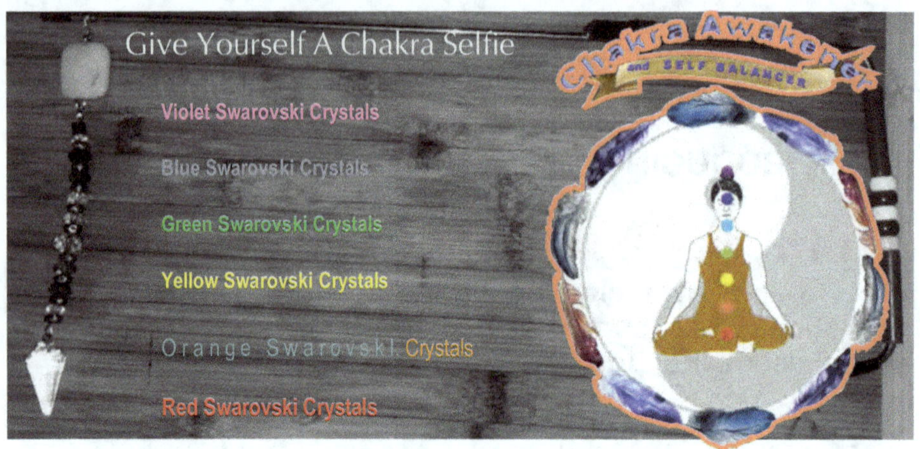

This beautifully hand-crafted **Chakra Awakener** is a powerful healing tool that gets rid of electromagnetic pollution (EMFs) in the subtle body. The charge from the crystal's magnetic energy changes the effect of the negativity and stress of this world.

The pendulum reads your body's energy as it gyrates around the chakra. For most Source Believers, test to find out which direction is right for you. May rotate opposite way. (You can use pendulum separately.)

- *Even movement in a clockwise direction indicates balance.*
- *Counterclockwise indicates imbalance.* (May be opposite)
- *Back and forth means blocked energy.*

Important Note:

Please Note: It's essential to cleanse and energize your stones and crystals as soon as you obtain them. Allow them to sit-in salt for 20 minutes, or sage them or use Crystal bowls for the best results once a week.

Exercise #2 Breathing and doing Affirmations; Take a deep breath through your nose instead of your mouth while focusing on drawing air into your chest first, then into your lower rib area, and finally into your lower belly. Do affirmation for the day of area, and finally into your lower belly. Do affirmation for the day of the week while focusing on the color of the chakra. (See page 42)

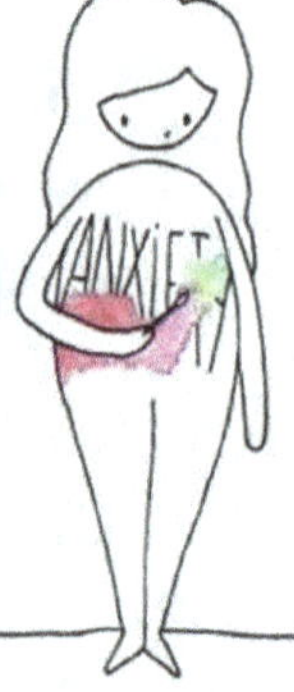

How to Give Yourself a Chakra Selfie

How to give yourself a Chakra Selfie

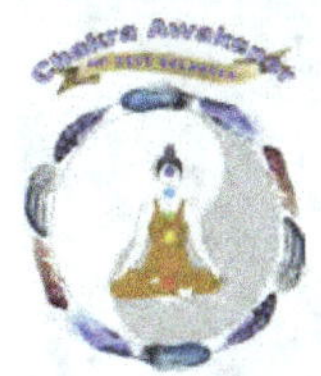

This is the fun part, the chakra awakener will auto-magically go to the chakra that needs balancing the most first, usually it's the Heart Chakra.

Lay down in a comfortable position, without crossing your legs. Get a small pillow to put under your arm, if needed. (Use your Zen oils and massage onto the chakras before using your Chakra Awakener.)

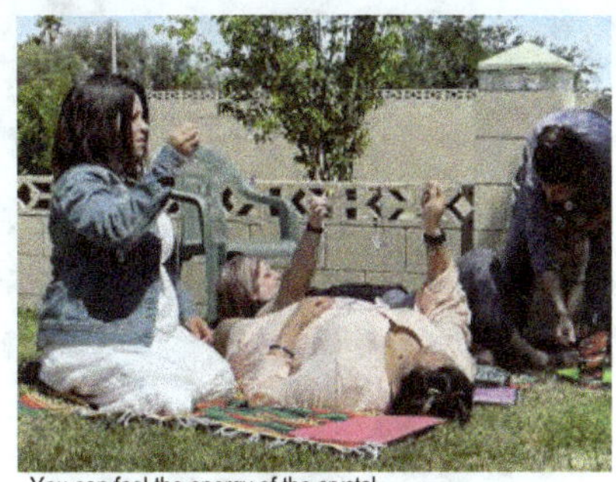
You can feel the energy of the crystal.

You may need to use a pillow for arm support

How to Meditate with your Chakra Selfie Stick

Use your intuition and feel the energy of the crystals.

While proceeding to each Chakra feel the presence of the Chakra within you.

Meditate and move your consciousness into that 'wheel' or energy center of your body.

Meditate on the issue within that Chakra by expanding it as much as is comfortable and then feel the crystals. Crystals are pure, if you can feel the nature or pure vibrations of the crystal and you can match your own frequency to it you are clearing or unlocking that Chakra. We want to make them all the same size.

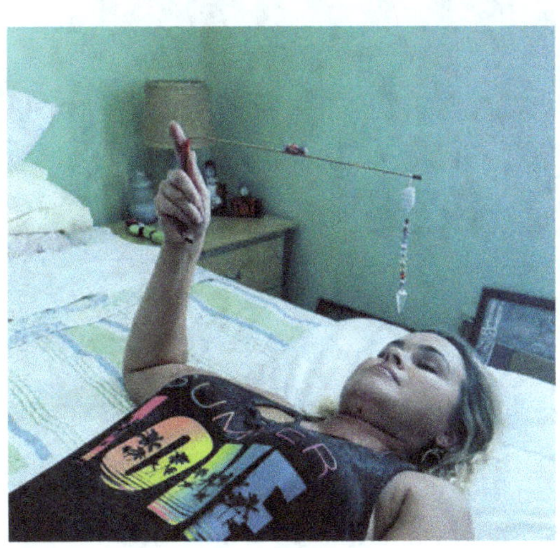

The Chakra Awakener can channel healing energy into your Chakras to restore frequency into your body and bring your *Spirit* back to good health.

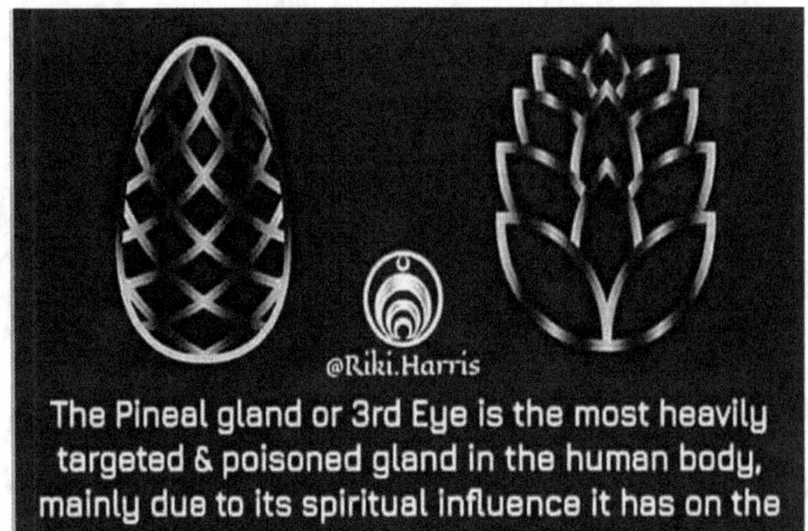

photo by @Riki.Harris

Morphogenetic Chakra work

Together as energy wheels. If one Chakra is imbalanced or blocked, it spreads to the others and affects your overall health and ability to function at the highest possible vibe.

All your Chakras need to be aligned and working in perfect health. To practice opening your third eye.

How to Give Yourself a Chakra Selfie

After you give yourself a Chakra Selfie - Aligning your chakras

TO GET RID OF NEGATIVE ENERGY -**YOU MUST**…
- Purge it out of your physical, emotional, and mental bodies.
- Use mantras, mudras, yoga, affirmations, crystals, oils, herbs, chinese medicine, self-love, and **Crystal Sound Therapy**.
- Let all that doesn't serve you, go!

Start by placing your hands on your Chakras. Place your left hand on your root chakra, right hand on the Sacral Chakra. While your right hand is on your Sacral Chakra, slowly move it to your Heart Chakra. Then do alternating hands on each Chakra.

Your Left hand is your receiving hand, and your right hand is your giving hand.

- *Move your hand in a clockwise direction starting at your belly button.*
- *Do Reiki symbols over each Chakra. (if you are attuned)*
- *Put hands together over the heart Chakra pause, give thanks.*
- *Place corresponding stones on Chakras- *Leave on the 5-30 minutes.*

Important Note:

Chakras shrink when we think fearful thoughts and enlarge out of balance when we become obsessed. *When you feel a need to remove the crystals then place a crystal pyramid on each chakra to release trapped energy. Leave on for however long you feel needed.

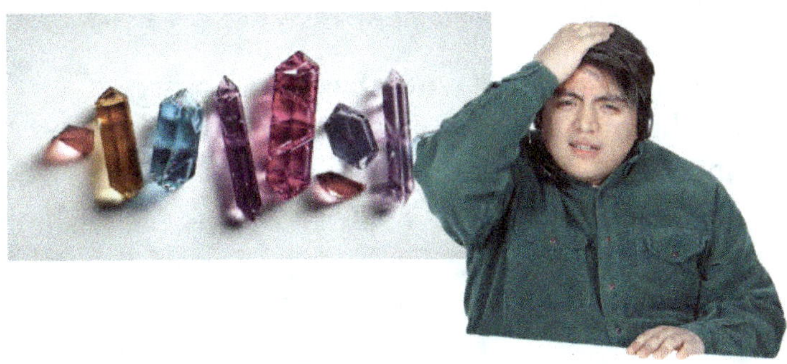

Particle Wave Chakras

There are seven progressive layers for each Chakra, each progressive layer Is a higher frequency like in a rainbow.

The pathways are sealed in most people, they open through the intention to align, while expanding their consciousness or through spiritual purification work.

(Illustration B)

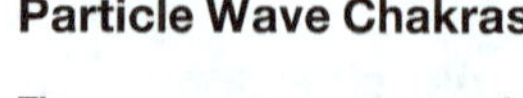

(Illustration C)

Auric Layers

Chakra balancing should be a part of your daily routine, like exercising and eating right , as our chakras need continuous fine-tuning.

If you are starting with chakra cleansing, it is helpful to begin with your root chakra and work your way up.

The Bodies

Location of your Chakras

on your Biological Clothing

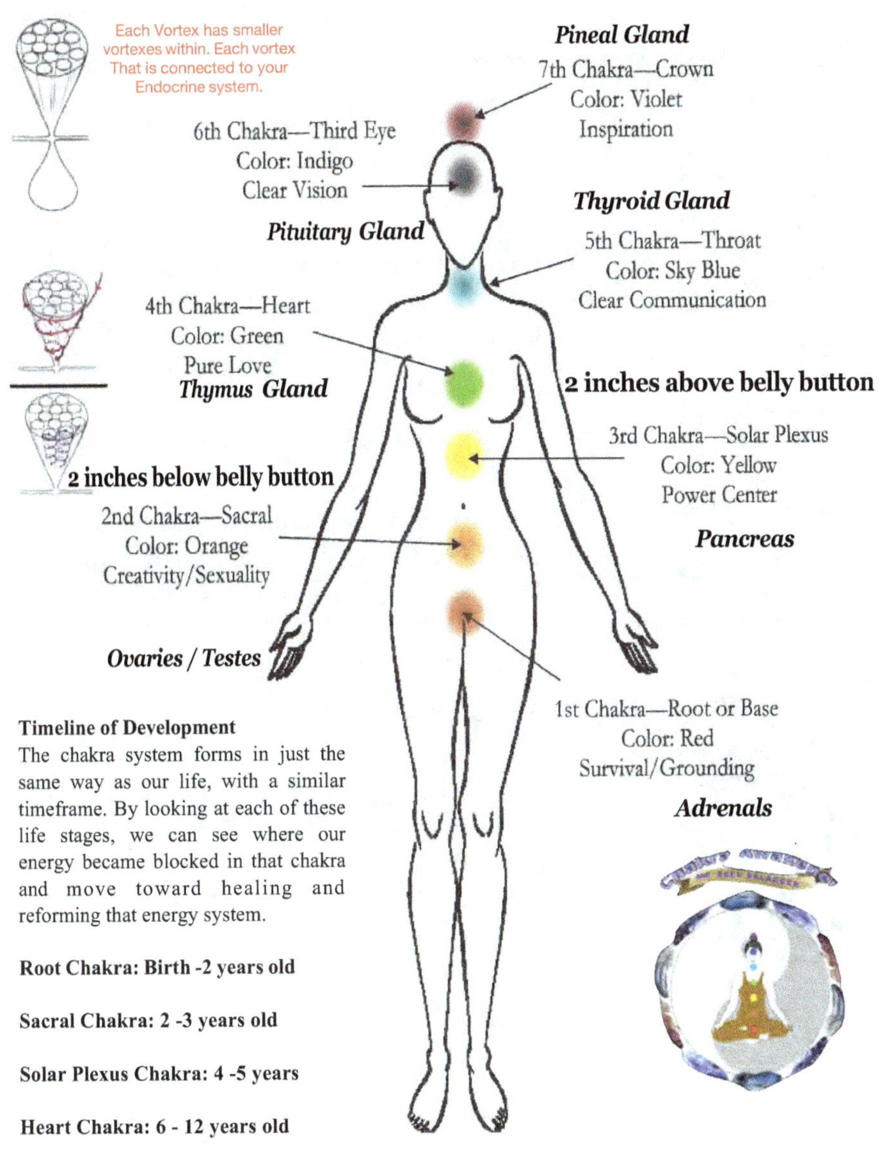

Timeline of Development
The chakra system forms in just the same way as our life, with a similar timeframe. By looking at each of these life stages, we can see where our energy became blocked in that chakra and move toward healing and reforming that energy system.

Root Chakra: Birth -2 years old

Sacral Chakra: 2 -3 years old

Solar Plexus Chakra: 4 -5 years

Heart Chakra: 6 - 12 years old

Throat Chakra: 13 - 19 years old

How to Give Yourself a Chakra Selfie

Looking for ways to make energy health a focus in your daily life? You can achieve physical wellness, mental clarity, and spiritual balance today.

Let's Get Started...

Play music - Chakra Bliss

You can download from **www.Ascensions.us/chakraselfie**

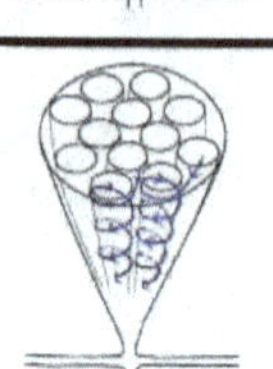

To start, take 3 Deep Breaths -

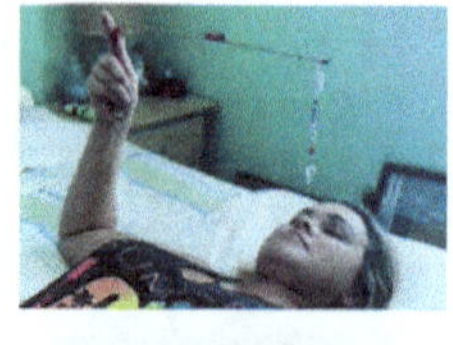

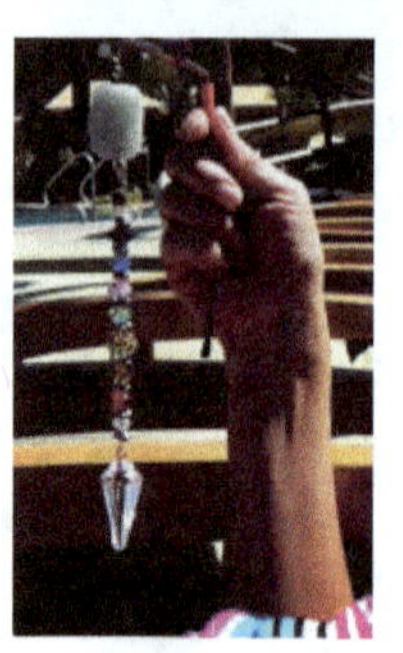

1. **Focus** on each bead starting at the bottom.
2. **Visualize** each bead's color, which is the color of the chakra, as the crystal is spinning; visualize the chakra color.
3. **Visualize** each color, 3-5 breaths (while listening to music that lasts about 15 minutes.)
4. ***Start at Root*** - *Red,* **Sacral** - *Orange,*
5. **Solar Plexus** - *Yellow* **Heart** - *Green and Pink,* **Throat** - *Blue,* **Crown** - *Violet.*
6. *1 min* **each then build up to** *3 minutes or more*
7. *Add specific types of Crystals to Chakras for certain effects.*

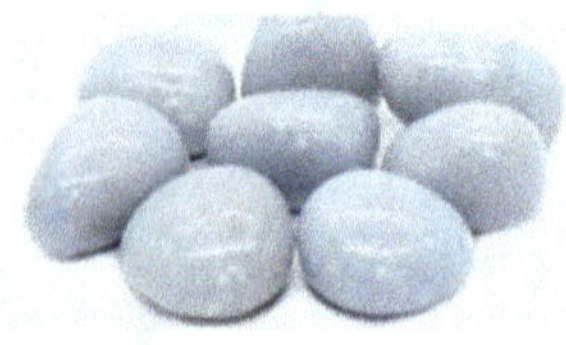

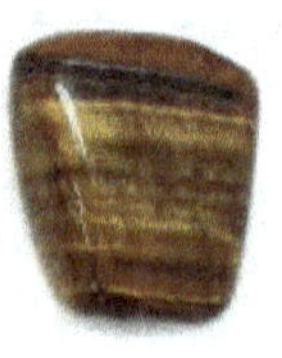

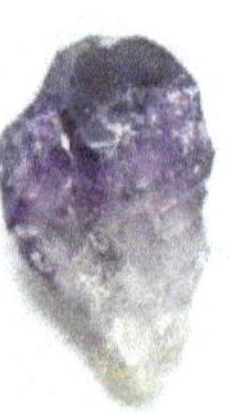

Give Yourself A Chakra Selfie Daily

Chakra Awakener is beneficial & necessary to grow the 'new skin' required to expand you into a higher frequency and multidimensionality. To accelerate this process. The Chakra awakener is a virtual accelerator that aids you in your metamorphosis and prepares you for the heightened energies of the ascension that you seek in the biological clothing that you temporarily wear.

In the sub-conscious MIND, not the ego-brain, is your greater identity. Know that you are in physical reality to master the lessons of the physical duality world.

There is a process occurring within your body (biological clothing) that is a microcosm in the macrocosm, and that needs to be understood. Our entire planet is quickening, to increase in frequency, you must ready yourselves to contain that frequency. If you are experiencing this stretching and building of this what they call 'new auric skin', you are going through an *Auric Metamorphosis.*

Auric Metamorphosis or *Changing of the Etheric Skin* as they call it, some of you are going though periods of depression; you feel as though you are sinking into a funk, and it seems like you are moving through molasses. Emotions go from ecstatic highs to deep lows shadowed in dark despair. If the damage is not recognized and reconciled, it can lead to chronic polarity reversal, emotional lows, depression, chronic fatigue syndrome, insomnia, migraines, weight gain, anxiety and panic disorders to list but a few.

The result is that your inner EMF is pulling in great surges of energy, energy levels that are somewhat greater than the parameters of your auric capacitors. In these cases, the result is that of stretching, an overload occurs resulting in temporary fissure cracks and energy loss. You may hear ringing in the ears.

Part of this metamorphic stretching requires a cleansing process. The very multidimensionality of chakras and of the Ascension itself are 'crucibles' and will force one's issues to the surface, and thus allow the entity a vital opportunity to confront & release any embedded obstacles. Better now than later. This is why they keep popping up for so many of you. Attempts to re-bury them, ignoring them will merely cause the issues to grow, fester and pop up again . These issues themselves, unresolved, will generate stress, and lead to the reactive fields of polar reversal and auric bleeding.

**Add specific crystals on the Chakras for more intense
clearing; crystals amplify one's energy field and help hold it intact.**

Identifying Your Behaviors

When we are in ***Energetic Balance*** with ourselves, we are in balance with our ***Spiritual Self,*** *balanced in* our emotional heart, and we cease to have great personal turmoil and suffering from our egoic-mind. (*An aspect of the mind that is not useful but pretends to be useful*) Then we become increasingly healthy and peaceful. When we are emotionally healthy and peaceful, we can easily access our spiritual self and heart intelligence.

The goal is to identify and locate these spiritually abusive behaviors in your Self, based on the Law of One. **The Law of One** is the **Universal Truth that All Is One -** in Spirit, so we can all relate.

Ascension, also known as Spiritual Awakening, is a simultaneous increase of *Expanding Consciousness* that occurs when our spiritual-energetic bodies, connect into our physical bodies. When our Chakras are blocked, it is more challenging to make the connection.

IDENTIFY BEHAVIORS

1. **Disassociation and Narcissism** - Crown Chakra Blocked
2. **Mental Rigidity** - Third Eye Blocked
3. **Emotional Fracturing** - Heart Chakra Blocked
4. **Carelessness** - Crown Chakra Blocked
5. **Deceitfulness** - Throat and Crown Blocked
6. **Dependence** - Sacral Chakra Blocked
7. **Service to Self** - (Ego) Root Chakra Blocked
8. **Divided Competition** (Ego) Root Chakra Block

*Watch out for **Service to Self**-games from others; it is when a predator liar gives disinformation. This person will try to gain an advantage over others, giving them the illusion that they will be greatly rewarded on the material plane. Ego is the resistance, of what is causing the negative energy.*

How to Give Yourself a Chakra Selfie
EMOTIONAL SOURCES OF DISEASE

This is just some of the emotional sources of Dis-ease and what crystal helps with healing. To find out more join our classes. ascensions.us/classes

Problem	*Source/Crystals to use*
Accidents	Expressions of anger, frustration, rebellion. **Blue Lace Agate**, **Moss Agate.**
Anorexia	Self-hate, denial of life nourishment, "not good enough". **Ocean Jasper, Bloodstone**
Arms	Ability to embrace, old emotions held in joints. **Jasper, Aquamarine**
Arthritis	Pattern of criticism of self & others, perfectionism. **Fluorite, Amethyst, Garnet**
Asthma	Smother-love, guilt complex, inferiority complex. **Emerald, Peridot, Tourmaline**
Back	Upper – not feeling supported emotionally, needing support. **Rose quartz, Chrysoprase** Middle – guilt. **Amber, Sodalite** Lower – burnout, worrying about money. **Carnelian.**
Breasts	Mothering, over-mothering a person/thing/place/experience. Breast cancer: deep resentment. Attached to over-mothering. **Amethyst, Carnelian, Clear Quartz, & Rose Quartz**

<h1 style="text-align:center">How to Give Yourself a Chakra Selfie</h1>

Clearing and Activating Chakras

Play music - https://youtu.be/b7JS0O3pFS8

Reiki Healing Music Can be download from www.Ascensions.us/chakraselfie

Quick Chakra Tune-up by Meditative Mind

Check out our meditation page.

Put the Chakra Balancer pendulum over the desired Chakra you're trying to balance and charge. Focus on your Chakra to be calibrated. To make this Chakra alignment, you must focus on the Chakra's color and the placement of the Chakra. To help you focus on the color, look at the beads on the pendulum. *(see chart, Pg. 19*

Once the Chakra Balancer stops over your desired Chakra, try and hold it there until the pendulum stops spinning. Close your eyes, take a few deep breaths for about 30 seconds then change hands. Move to the next Chakra and do it over again.

7   ways to clearing and activating the Main Chakras:

1. Open, clear, and balance the grounding energy

of the first Chakra by visualizing tree roots.

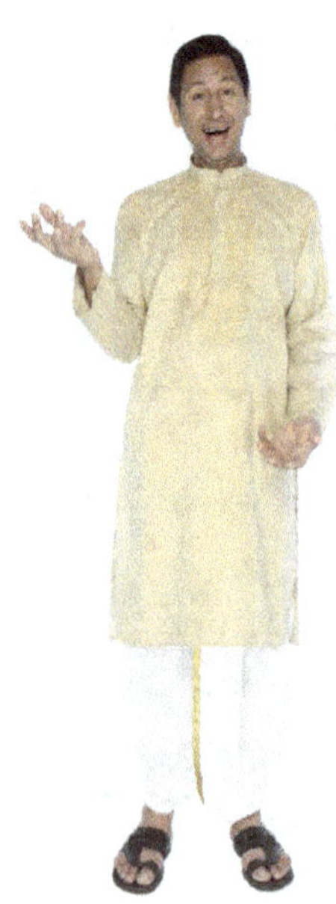

- **2. Vibrationally stimulate** the second Chakra with tuning forks.
- **3.Recharge** the self-empowerment that resides in the 3rd Chakra.
- **4.Re-connect** with the nurturing unconditional Love that you are, which is anchored in your heart. Open your heart Chakra.
- **5. Open** the channels of communication connecting you with all of life's gifts by clearing the fifth Chakra.
- **6. Open** your power of eternal vision by activating the 6th, Chakra.
- **7. Enhance** your oneness with Divinity by Clearing and energizing the 7th Crown Chakra.

How to Give Yourself a Chakra Selfie

Your aura is the energy field that surrounds your entire body.

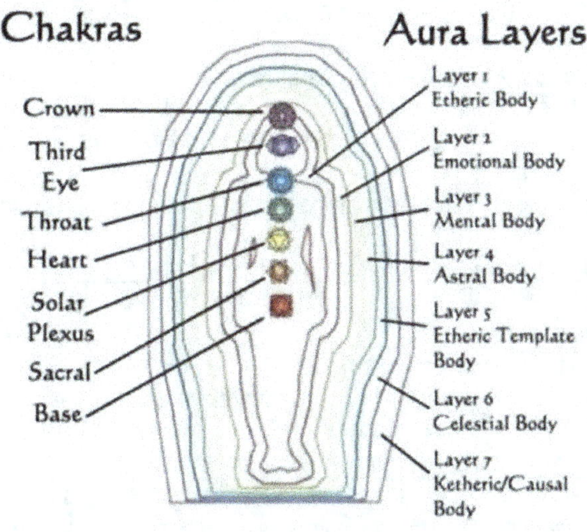

Connected to the seven energy centers of the chakras is your Aura, which is comprised of 7 different layers. Each layer will vary in depth and size, depending on the person and where they are on their spiritual path. In a healthy state, the entire Aura can extend several feet from the physical body and is very bright. In an unhealthy state, the auric field can be small and dull. The odd-numbered layers tend to be more structured and carry a yang type of energy, whereas the even layers are more fluid and carry a Yin type of energy.

1st Auric Layer is Etheric.
- Closest to the physical body
- Represents the physical body, muscles, tissues, bones, etc.
- Connected to the root chakra
- A bluish color
- Easiest to see with the naked eye
- Stronger in athletes and those who are very active
- Weaker in those who lead a sedentary lifestyle or when immunity is compromised

2nd Auric Layer: Emotional - Second from the physical body

- Represents emotions and feelings
- Connected to the **Sacral Chakra**
- Can be muddy colored during times of emotional stress
- State of the chakras can be easily determined from this layer

3rd Auric Layer: Mental - Third from the physical body

- Represents thoughts, cognitive processes and state of mind
- Bright yellow in color
- Connected to the **Solar Plexus Chakra**
- Often radiates the strongest around the head, neck and shoulders
- Stronger in those who engage in mental tasks or those who have an over-active mind
- When engaging in a creative activity, colored sparks can also be seen flowing from this layer

4th Auric Layer: Astral - Fourth from the physical body

- Represents where we form our astral cords with others
- Pink or rosy in color
- Connected to the heart chakra
- Becomes stronger through loving, intimate relationships
- Can be weaker during breakups or conflicts with loved ones

5th Auric Layer: Etheric Template - Fifth from the physical body

- Represents the entire blueprint of the body that exists on this physical plane
- Includes everything you create on this physical level including your identity, personality and overall energy
- Connected to the throat chakra
- Can vary in color usually, blue
- Healed and made stronger by expressing your truth and knowing who you truly are

6th Auric Layer: Celestial - Sixth from the physical body

- Connected to the third eye chakra
- Carries a very strong and powerful vibration
- Represents the connection to the Divine and all other beings
- Where unconditional love and feelings of oneness flow
- Pearly white in color
- When strong, the person may have the ability to communicate with the spirit world and receive angelic messages
- Can be healed with unconditional love

7th Auric Layer: Ketheric Template - Seventh from the physical.

- Furthest away from the physical body (estimated around 2-3 ft. away)
- Represents the feeling of being one with the Universe
- Holds all the information about your soul and previous lifetimes
- Vibrates at the highest frequency
- Connected to the crown chakra
- Gold in color

How to Give Yourself a Chakra Selfie

Your Electromagnetic Field

The auric field or human electromagnetic field requires a particular physical, mental, and emotional well-being to operate the whole circuitry to ensure one's growth and prosperity. Dysfunction in any of these areas can create an effect called auric bleeding. It will cause short circuitry that generates varying levels of detrimental energy loss through 'auric fissuring,' leading to an energetic downward spiral.

The Human Auric Field is not auto regulated; it requires maintenance. It flows optimally encased in an oval sheath and is maintained at a specific circuitry balance. Understanding the mechanics of the Aura is requisite for humanity in the energy of the New Earth of 2020 and beyond. For the past 15 millennia, the Aura has coordinated through the electromagnetic grid in linear terms. It has been (up until 2012) the electromagnetic grid that all forms of the earth-plane of life were projected. Everything on our planet is composed of energy, and all energy is alive, even from what you term as inanimate objects.

As the 144-Crystalline grid completed in 2012, the Human Aura transitioned and is yet shifting into a Crysto-Electrical field. This Crysto-Electrical field has been ongoing for several years, since what is termed the initial phase of the Cosmic Trigger. The new Crysto-Electrical Field is composed of 12 physio layers, with each physio CEF layer having its own function or role. An aura is not separate from the physical body but is an extension of it in different ethereal compositions.

Understanding the workings of your Auric Field and the auric expansion, while using the Chakra Balancer is why you may be experiencing what is known as Ascension Maladies or Ascension Symptoms. Because, when you are trying to maintain your emotions. (a.k.a. Energy in motion). You must also learn to maintain your auric field. When your auric field is short-circuited, or energy is lost, you will have emotional extremes, from high to low, which can occur up until the time that the imbalanced auric field is re-stabilized, re-balanced & re-grounded.

Sometimes with pharmaceuticals, or you may utilize pure sonic frequency thru crystal bowls, Tibetan bowls & tuning forks. (See page 34) Now, in addition to this, be aware of your emotional state. Suppose you are suffering from lethargy, chronic fatigue, insomnia, depression, and anxiety. It will undoubtedly serve you to take the steps listed in the booklet, but other actions will likely be required. Depending on how far along you are in your dis-ease.

How to Give Yourself a Chakra Selfie

ASCENSION ENERGY

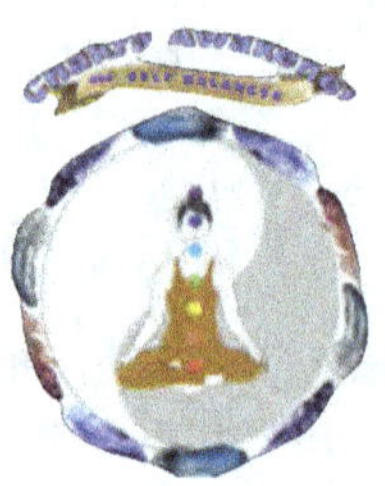

Regarding Ascension, one of the most important concepts for you to understand and accept is the fact that everything in your reality is energy.

- Your soul is energy.

- You are made of Male & Female Spiritual Energy.

- Your physical body is made of electromagnetic energy.

- You are a unified energy system in which all parts are influencing each other.

- Matter is a manifestation of energy.

- There is no separation since everything in the Universe, including you, originates from the one Source. You are part and parcel of the One Source Energy.

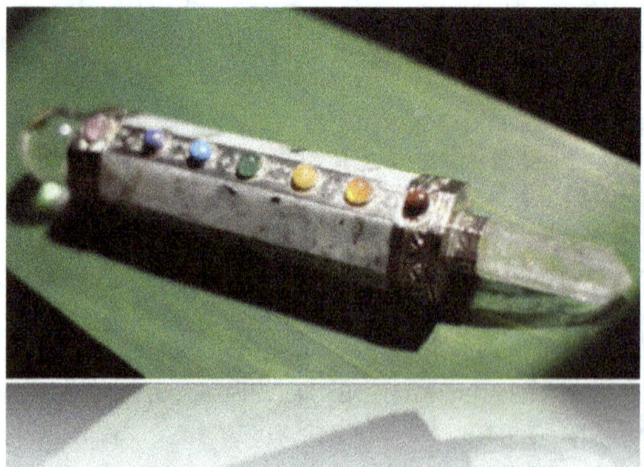

You can use Phi Vogel Crystals for strengthening the aura, and repairing fissures, along with using the Chakra Awakener every day.

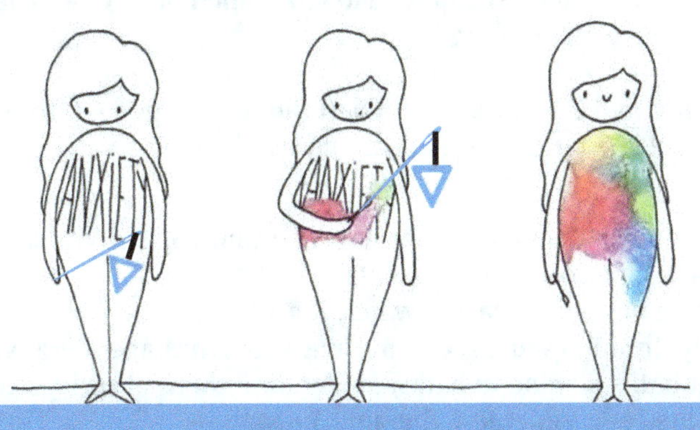

Exercise #3 FEEL YOUR EMOTIONS!

Practice for one week.

Then the obstacles to your purity will dissolve.

Clearing your Chakras is like pouring Caro syrup on your nerves. Every day, on the nightly news, we are bombarded with tragedies, our boss or co-workers upset us, a car cut us off.

We have been born into an electromagnetic soup that our ancestors couldn't have dreamed of, and our food and drink choices aren't the best; they are all the trappings of modern life that pollute our subtle energy bodies. <u>**See page 40**</u> to help eliminate stuck emotions.

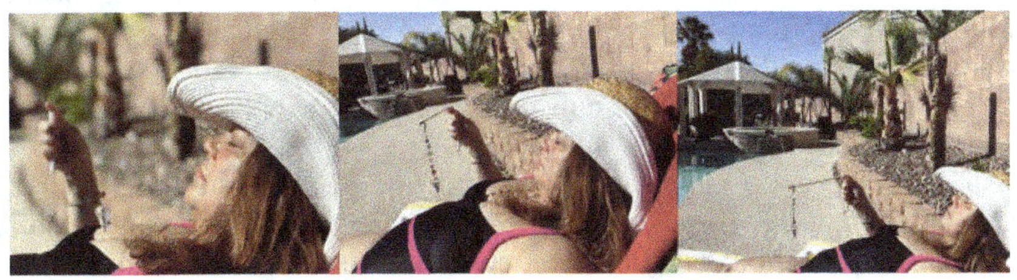

16 ways to raise your auric frequency quotient

You can reconcile these; first, you must ready yourselves to contain that frequency, by using the Chakra Awakener/ Selfie Balancer and learn how to determine your auric frequency.

Aspects of life that are worsened in part due to energy loss from the hectic pace of life by lack of exercise and an unhealthy diet.

1. Exercise at least 20 minutes per day. (Tai Chi, Yoga or Walking) 5 pts.
2. Increase water consumption. 5 pts
3. Magnetize or add crystals to water. 5 pts
4. Detoxify, through saunas, colonic irrigation, massage therapy. 5 pts
5. Use salt baths & mineral baths, and natural thermal springs. 5 pts
6. Utilize the Tesla Violet Ray Therapy. 5 pts
7. Use of magnetics on the soles of the feet & wrist 5 pts
8. Wear specific combinations of gemstones. 5 pts
9. Wear noble metal around the neck and on both wrists. 5 pts
10. Healthy diet. 5 pts
11. Avoid excess alcohol. 5 pts
12. Eliminate / minimize toxins, tobacco and certain prescription drugs. 5 pts
13. Take cleansers weekly such as garlic, ginger and Apple cider vinegar. 5 pts
14. Work with Phi cut Vogel crystals, in auric sealing, strengthening the aura, and repairing fissures. 5 pts
15. Smudge, sage the auric field. 5 pts
16. Utilize pure sonic frequency thru crystal bowls, Tibetan bowls & tuning forks. 5 pts

Now, in addition to this, be aware of your emotional state. If you are suffering from lethargy, chronic fatigue, insomnia, depression, and anxiety, it will undoubtedly serve you to take the steps listed above, but other actions will likely be required.

Many of you have chosen specific life lessons that involve removing obstacles in life by overcoming 'contractual set-ups.' These set-up life lessons are, in essence, opportunities and gifts if you will allow it to move you forward. Remember, If they were easy, you would not necessarily learn.

Wear a chain around the neck with a stabilizing pendant, such as lapis lazuli, malachite or azurite. Through this process, you have a more exceptional ability to increase your field and deflect opposing (negative energy attachments) energy fields, you see. Clear gems are great producers of higher dimensional light waves and amplify one's area and help to hold it intact.

Working Through Negativity
Questionnaire

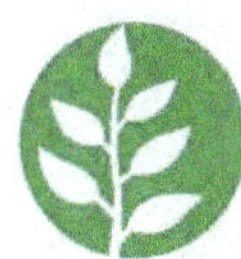

1. Are you an impatient person?

Yes ☐ No ☐   *Why?*

2. Do you create a life that doesn't support you being the best that you can be?

Yes ☐ No ☐   *Why?*

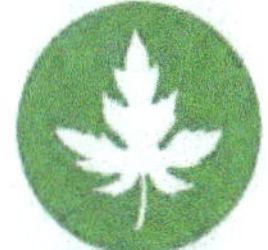

3. Do you have difficulty trying new things?

Yes ☐ No ☐   *Why?*

4. Do you have a loss of interest in socializing?

Yes ☐ No ☐   *Why?*

If you answered "Yes" to all the questions, then you have an under active Chakra. If you answered 1/2 "Yes" and 1/2 "No" Your Crown Chakra is out of balance. All "No's" You have learned to balance your Chakras.

How to Give Yourself a Chakra Selfie

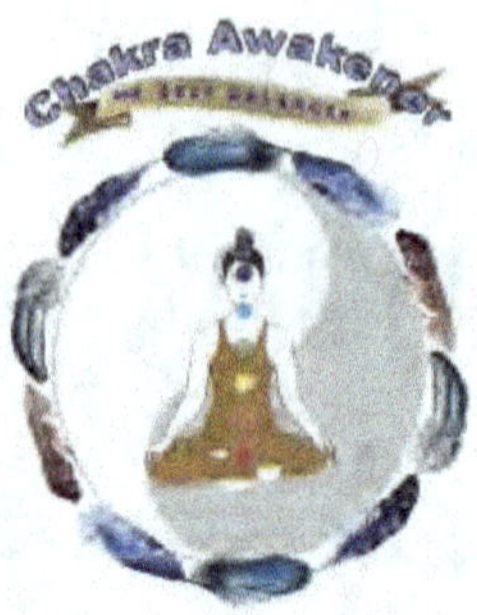

Under-Active Chakra Symptoms

There are many physical symptoms that you might experience that could indicate an under-active chakra: Here are a few…

- Nerve problems. This can often lead to numbness in your extremities and loss of dexterity.

- Muscular Atrophy. This means that muscles degenerate and weaken, which can in extreme circumstances leave you bedridden. – though by that point you should have seen a doctor.

- Various neurological conditions. The crown chakra is intricately linked with the brain and problems in the brain often stem from an under-active crown chakra.

- Dullness of the senses. Colors might seem less vivid, you might have trouble hearing things, and food can become tasteless and unappetizing.

- These physical symptoms can range in severity from the very mild to the immediately problematic.

- Severe health problems should always be referred to a doctor, just in case there is an underlying condition that is too far gone.

- Lack of purpose or direction in life. The crown chakra helps us to find the meaning in life, so when it is under-active, we might find ourselves struggling to see the point of it all.

- Loss of interest in socializing. Our sense of unity in the universe and with each other is rooted in the crown chakra, so under-activity affects our interest in being sociable.

- Depression. Chemical imbalances in the brain are often the cause of depression, and an imbalance in the crown chakra only exacerbates this.

How to Give Yourself a Chakra Selfie

• <u>Difficulty learning new skills</u> or taking on board new ideas. The crown chakra dramatically influences our thirst for knowledge, and when it is found lacking, we are less on the ball when it comes to new ideas.

• <u>Negative attitude or</u> pessimism. Some people are just pessimistic, but when someone does so in a way that is out of character for them it can usually be attributed to under-active crown chakra. So you've worked out whether or not you have an under-active crown chakra.

Healing an Under-Active Crown Chakra

The best way to heal an under-active crown chakra is through chakra healing meditation. In your quiet, spiritual place you should enter into a deep state of meditation as your practice allows.

Once there, while holding your *Chakra Awakener* you can move your focus up through your body, beginning at the root chakra at the base of the spine and moving up, finally finishing on the crown chakra at the top of your head.

See link on www.Ascensions.us/chakraselfie

Maintain this focus, but remain indifferent to what you experience. This is an observation stage, where you are zeroing in on the problem.

While holding the *Chakra Awakener* maintain focus as it moves across your body automatically. You may use a pillow under your arm for support.

After 3 minutes, you should begin visualization. Think of colors and images, visualizing the spiritual connections that link you to this world and the astral plane. Consider unity consciousness.

Then, as you pull out of the meditative state, allow yourself to relax into contemplation.

You can concentrate on your direction in life, the purpose you have chosen for yourself and how you will figure out your needs with the spiritual truths.

Start a journal, write it down.

Do this 3 or 4 times a week, and your crown chakra should start to find its balance. (for more chakra instruction go to **www.ascensions.us/ chakras)**

How to Give Yourself a Chakra Selfie

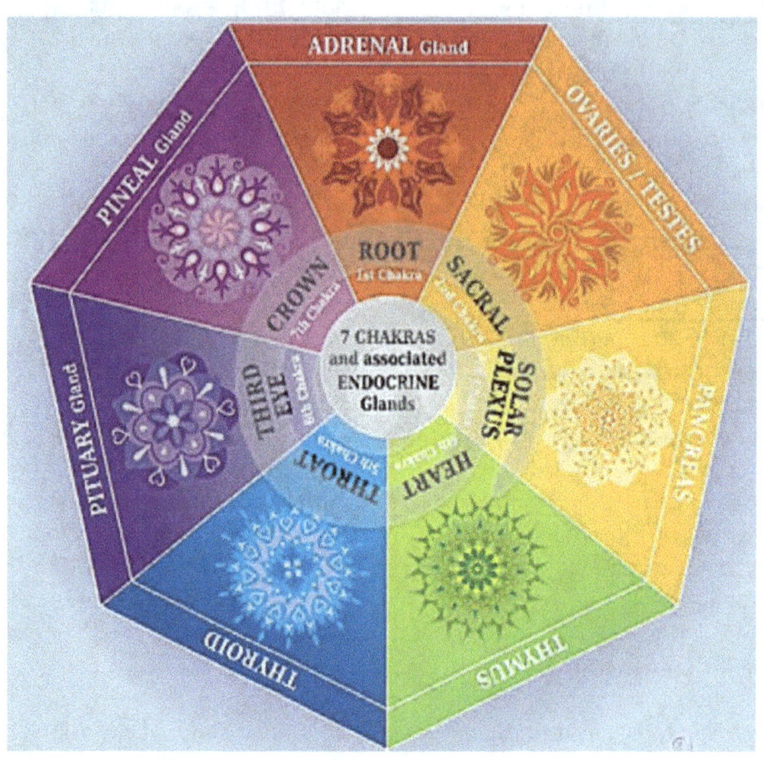

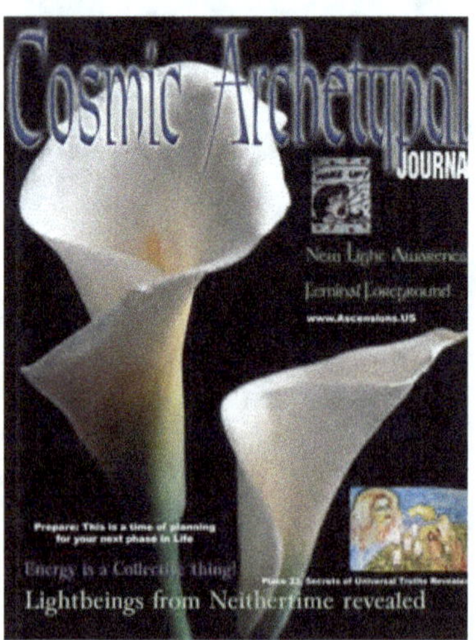

Order our monthly. Newsletter a t www.Ascensions.us.

Gain the understanding of the workings of your auric field and the auric expansion coming, and what may be termed as 'Ascension Maladies' or Ascension Symptoms. Maintaining your E-motions. (Energy in motion).

Frequency

**Utilize pure sonic frequency thru crystal bowls,
Tibetan bowls & tuning forks.**

Your Chakras are the energy centers of your body. If they aren't absorbing energy from the Universe, it will lead to illness, depression, pain, relationship issues, and more. Reiki is a holistic healing art from Japan that can channel healing energy into your Chakras to restore your body and spirit to good health. Learn self-Reiki or find a good practitioner.

What are Crystal Singing Bowls?

Singing Bowls produce a harmonization between their vibration and that of the person. Resonance is the principle on which vibrational medicine works. Resonance is the capacity of a particular wave to produce a response in something with a similar vibration. The vibration of Crystal bowls has the power to make atoms vibrate and reorganize themselves in a crystalline structure, which is stronger, healthier, and more balanced.

The sound will holistically affect the whole individual, balancing the energetic body and chakras and cleaning the auric field. The vibration spikes the spinal cord, acting as an energetic resonance vehicle sending the waves through the nervous system, cells, tissue, and organs. These tones or vibrations bring the individual playing or listening to heightened states of consciousness because of the effect on inter-neuron connections.

The sound waves produced by the bowls induce a state of relaxation like long-term meditation practice. While in this relaxed state caused by the bowls, the mind guides the consciousness on an inner journey giving the sensation of what Zen Masters call *"filling oneself up with emptiness."* This state of emptiness provides us with the opportunity to see the world and ourselves from a different perspective.

How will Singing Bowls make me feel?

The people who experience the effects of the bowls describe it as a deep physical and mental relaxation, sensations of floating, and wellbeing. The experience can unblock and dissolve energetic and physical obstructions in the physical and astral body, and this is a therapeutic tool for deep healing. Because the seven musical notes reverberate in the seven chakras, and the seven colors of the human aura create a vibrational bath that emits a natural balancing effect.

Placement of ionic generators, such as halite salt blocks and air filters, helps restore the anion to cation ratio in rooms containing computers, microwaves, and televisions. Book your appointment now!

 www.Ascensions.us

Oils for your Chakras

How do essential oils work?

Essential oils have been used medicinally for decades and shown to cleanse toxins from the body. They are also indicated to improve the ability of the body to absorb essential nutrients and vitamins. Essential oils can enter the body through skin application, ingestion, or inhalation (aromatherapy).

When applied to the skin, essential oils are absorbed and the active ingredients are used by the body for specific therapeutic treatment. For example, applying a blend of essential oil containing ginger is said to reduce arthritis pain and increase flexibility.

Ingesting or consuming essential oils is not recommended and advisable only under the care of a trained clinician or physician. Ingestion of essential oils may cause adverse health effects, including toxicity to the liver and kidneys, gastric upset, and contraindications when taking other medications.

The most popular way essential oils enter the body is by inhaling their aroma through the nose. This is also known as aromatherapy. Inhaling essential oils is said to positively affect the olfactory and limbic systems of the body. The olfactory system relates to all organs contributing to our sense of smell.

The limbic system, also known as our emotional brain directly affects our heart rate, blood pressure, stress levels, hormones, breathing, and memory. The active ingredients in some essential oils when inhaled are said to travel to the lungs and improve our respiratory system. According to other studies, inhaling essential oils has favorable physiological effects on the human body in general.

Other research has indicated the inhaled form of citrus essential oil promotes relaxation and spearmint oil acts as a bronchodilator. These findings have stimulated further research on how citrus and spearmint essential oils can benefit athletic performance.

How to Give Yourself a Chakra Selfie

CHAKRA BALANCING OILS

Crown - Frankincense, Camphor, Myrrh

Third Eye - Jasmine, Basil, Lemon, Camphor, and Eucalyptus.

Throat - Sandalwood, Cajeput, Bergamot, Lavender.

Heart - Rose oil, Saffron, Palma Rosa.

Solar Plexus - Davina Flower, Fennel, Champa Flower, Geranium, Jasmine, Lavender, and Sandalwood.

Sacral - Patchouli, Ylang-Ylang, Geranium, Palma Rosa, Lemon and Neroli.

Root - Vetiver, Sandalwood, Cedar-wood, and Ginger.

Balance your physical body to become a Divine Human.

Order Oils & learn how to use the oils to go.
www.ascensions.us/oils.

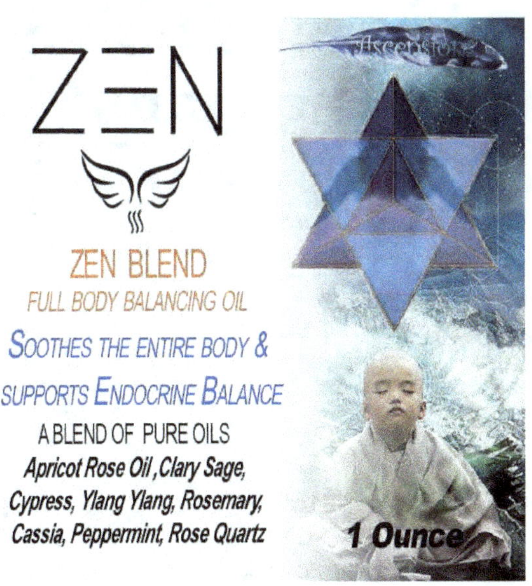

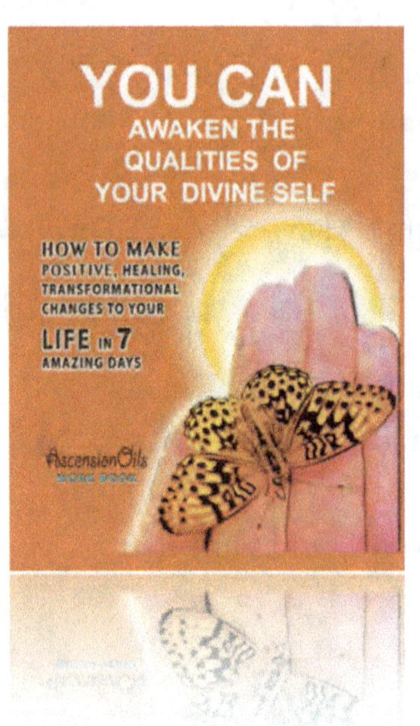

Hi, I'm here to help you overcome challenges, raise your vibration with the shifting of your consciousness, and show you how to gain new focus in your life to find your purpose and follow your bliss.

This information comes from the *Source*. *Our* mission is to learn how to become a forgiven soul.

Access powerful **Spiritual Light** To assist the evolution of others and the **Earth Mother** herself. To progress the Evolution of **Truth Seekers** and help people realize that we are all limitless beings. To expand our understanding of reality, share the truth of who we are, and assist people in aligning themselves consciously with **Universal Consciousness,** we must realize that Unity is the Truth of Oneness.

Your E-motions can harm your bodies organs!

Anger: **Weakens the Liver**

Grief: **Weakens the Lungs**

Worry: **Weakens the Stomach**

Stress: **Weakens the Heart & Brain**

Fear: **Weakens the Kidneys**

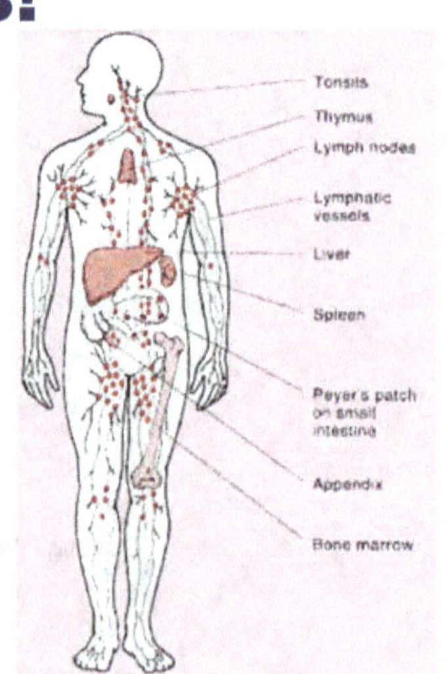

VERITAS - True Source Self Connection Pendulums at Ascensions.us

Veritas Pendulums can check your vital organs:

Who's using it ?

Summer- I had really bad anxiety and a friend recommended this balancer because it helped with her anxiety, I was extremely surprised by how well it worked in calming me with 5 kids in the house."

Shelley -You can do it anywhere! The colored crystals help you to visualize the chakra colors. I like doing it on the beach.

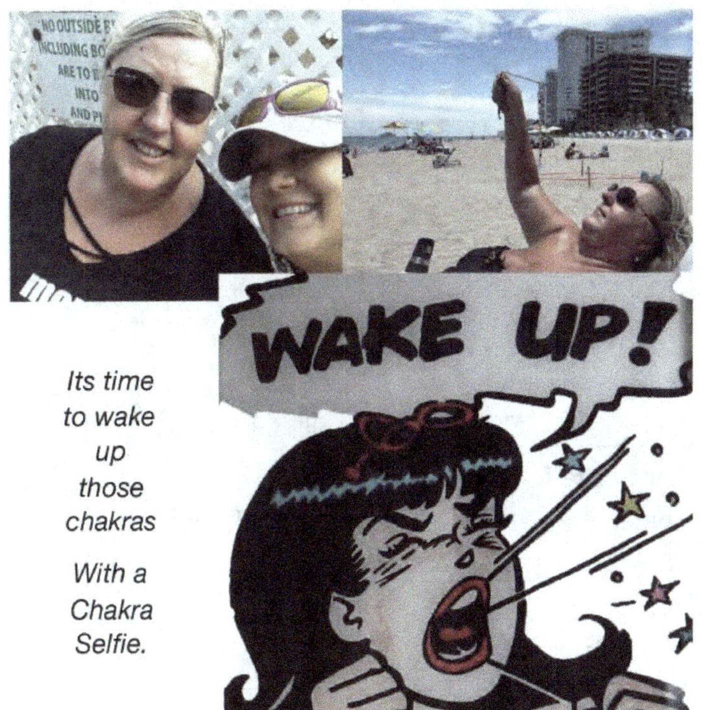

*Its time
to wake
up
those
chakras*

*With a
Chakra
Selfie.*

Photo -By Levi Bunnell

L.I.F.E. Living In Frequency Earth

How to Give Yourself a Chakra Selfie

Excessive Chakra Energy

Demanding

Overly critical

Tense between shoulders

Possessive

Moody

Melodramatic

Manic Depressive

Martyr Attitude

Conditional Love

Deficient Chakra Energy

Feels sorry for oneself

Paranoid

Indecisive

Afraid of

Letting go

Being free

Getting hurt

Being abandoned

Sexual energy:

Feels unworthy of love

Can't reach out

Needs constant reassurance

Antidote for balancing Chakra Energy

Green or Pink Crystals

By doing the _"Seven-day Mental Diet"_ to remove negative energy within your

*biofield, then sending it to the Earth for transmutation to positive energy you will be helping yourself become whole.

Email me for information.

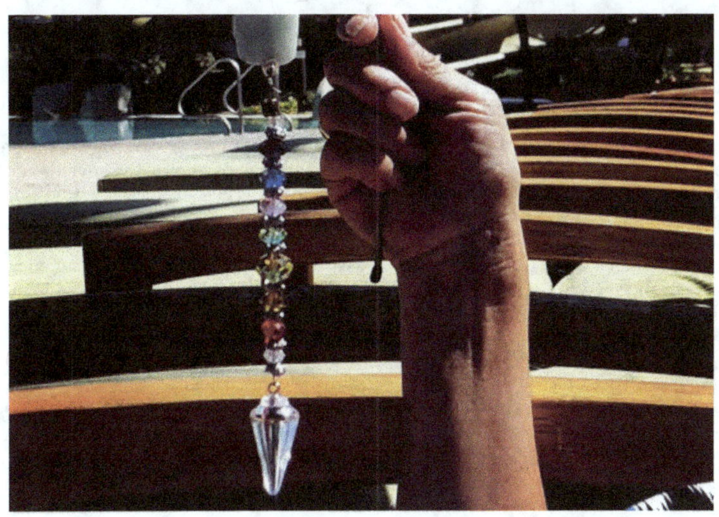

**Remember each chakra has vortexes of
energy spinning through them.**

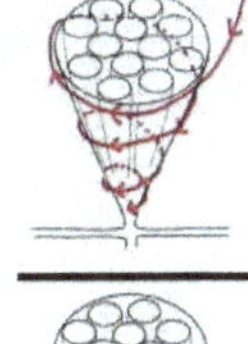
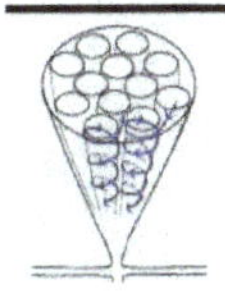

The energy also flows through the very fabric of the universe, also known as chi or Prana-energy. The energy system is blocked by emotional energy known as Cah.   Each day allow yourself to start in increments to let go of negative, Cah. In the beginning, it may be painful, to experience every drop of fluid negative Cah energy that you're damming up because you are not used to feeling your feelings.

Each Chakra governs a specific kind of energy-related to various human attributes and your endocrine system (See page 34).

When all Chakras are functioning well, we are healthy in body, mind, and spirit.

Prana is **an energy that pulses through the body along a network of subtle body channels**. Similar to the central nervous system, the channels of the subtle body, or nadis, connect form and mind and act as a conduit for energy.

Chakra balancer Affirmations

Affirmations from Adama -From the Seven Sacred Flames by Aurelia.
The Seven Rainbow Flames

Currently, I want to give you a short overview of the seven major rays. It would be very beneficial for each of you to focus each day on the energies of one of the seven major rays that flood the planet from Creator Source on that day. All energies of the seven rays flood the planet daily, but each day of the week, one of the rays becomes predominant.

Working with the seven rays in this manner will assist you, in a most profound way, to balance the energies of the seven rays in each one of your chakras throughout your life and will bring you much greater balance and grace. In the process of ascension and enlightenment, all seven major rays and later, the five Secret Rays, must be balanced and mastered in order to move on to greater wisdom and mastery in your cosmic future.

In Telos, we work much more effectively each day by amplifying in our hearts, our minds and our daily activities the specific energies of each day of the week. We invite you to experiment with this. You may be pleasantly surprised to discover how much more effectively the energies are amplified and how they assist you.

Sunday, the Yellow Ray of Wisdom, Illumination and the Mind of God is amplified. Focus on the Mind of God daily in all things, but specifically on Sunday. The Divine Mind will open your own mind to ever expanding Wisdom. True wisdom always comes from the mind of higher perspective and consciousness. As you
merge this divine mind with your own, you begin to make decisions and conduct your life in ways that will bring you much ease and satisfaction.

Monday, the Royal Blue Ray of the Will of God is amplified.
Focus on the Will of God for your very life through total surrender to that Divine Will, no matter what your present circumstances appear to be. This is the fastest way to gain your spiritual mastery and freedom. As you align with God's Will, you will notice that your life will manifest more harmony. Bathe your mind, body and soul each day with that energy, and soon, you will reap its many benefits.

Tuesday, the Rose-Pink Ray of Divine Love of God is amplified.
Focus on the transforming and healing influence of the energies of Divine Love. Love is the glue that creates, transforms, heals and harmonizes all things. Take time in your life to breathe it in and merge with this Flame of Divine Love, the key to the power of multiplication and all good things you desire. As you merge with this Flame in a greater measure, limitations start dissolving and you become the master of your destiny.

Wednesday, the Emerald Green Ray of the Divine Flame of Healing, Precipitation and Abundance is amplified. Focus on the energies of divine healing in all aspects of your life. This is a balancing and soothing energy that will assist you to align the many distortions you have created in your lives. Invoke and visualize this radiant green liquid healing light blazing through all areas where transformation is needed. The Green Ray also governs the laws of abundance and prosperity. Also invoke the emerald, green Flame to pave the way for the manifestation and precipitation of all your physical and spiritual desires

How to Give Yourself a Chakra Selfie

Thursday, the Golden Ray
Focus on the energies of this Flame for the resurrection and restoration of your inherited divinity. You are a divine being experiencing human life and learning from it. Because you have strayed in consciousness, your divinity has been veiled. As you invoke and merge with the purple and gold energies of the Resurrection Flame, you will start resurrecting all the gifts and attributes of your divinity. Along with the Violet Flame, this wondrous flame prepares you for the final ritual of Ascension, which is the main purpose for your many incarnations on this planet.
of the Resurrection Flame is amplified.

Friday, the Pure Dazzling White Ray of Purity *of the Ascension Flame is amplified. Ascension is the alchemical marriage or divine union of your human-self with your I AM Presence through the process of purification of all mis-qualification of God's energy throughout your many incarnations. Focus on purifying and clearing all negativity, false beliefs, poor attitudes and habits blocking the manifestation of your spiritual mastery.*

Saturday, the Penetrating Violet Ray of Transmutation *and Freedom is amplified. On Saturday, focus on the many tones and frequencies of the Violet Ray which is most magical. The Violet Flame brings the frequency of change, alchemy, freedom from limitations, royalty, diplomacy, comfort and much more. As you fill your auric field and your heart with the wonders of this Flame, its frequency will start clearing from your life the obstacles and karma that are obstructing the way to the realization of your mastery. Use the Violet Fire as much as you can each day, but especially on Saturday when this ray is amplified in a greater way, and it will serve you well.*

Fill your auric field and every cell of your physical, mental, emotional and etheric bodies with this pure-white dazzling Ascension Flame. In your meditation, do this with all the rays. It is essential for your spiritual progress.

As you see, my dear friends, all the rays are important. None of them can be neglected nor put aside. They all work together in perfect harmony to assist the restoration of your soul and Self-realization. Spiritual progress is brought forth as the result of daily application of God's Laws, God's energies through the seven main rays, and the clearing of one's karma and emotional body.

Each day, it is most important that you set time aside to do your spiritual work. Invoking the Sacred Flames and their attributes opens the channels to receive deeper understanding of cosmic laws. Breathe, invoke and fill yourself with these wondrous energies.

In your meditation, connect with the energy of these Flames as you contact your Divine Essence and your guides, diligently applying what is shown to you. Seek to lift the veil of mortal illusions and reconnect with the magic and power of the original intent of God for your eternal journey into greater purpose and destiny. Our assistance is also available to you for the asking; a simple prayer request from your heart brings us into your forcefield instantly in answer to your call.

Bloodstone Chakra Healing and Balancing Energy

Bloodstone is an intense healing stone used to cleanse and realign the lower chakras with the heart, and is conducive to balancing the total body in order to overcome any distress or anxiety associated with re-alignment of these energies. This stone is particularly stimulating to the Base and Heart Chakras.

The Base, or Root Chakra, is located at the base of the spine, and controls the energy for kinesthetic feeling and movement. It is the foundation of physical and spiritual energy for the body. When physically out of balance the symptoms manifest themselves as lethargy, low levels of activity, low enthusiasm, and a need for constant stimulation. When spiritual energies are out of balance, one may feel flighty, disconnected from reality or distant. Red crystal energy is used to clear blockages and re-balance the Base Chakra. In balance, the physical body regains its strength and stamina, and the spiritual energy is rekindled in the form of security and sense of one's own power. It often leads to independence and spontaneous leadership.

The Heart Chakra, located near the center of the breastbone, regulates our interaction with the external world and controls what we embrace and what we resist. It gives us the balancing ability to be ourselves within the environment. When the Heart Chakra is out of balance we may feel either controlling or controlled in a relationship, and become critical of the little foibles of others. We may find ourselves having inappropriately strong emotional responses to everyday external stimuli.

I Am Balanced

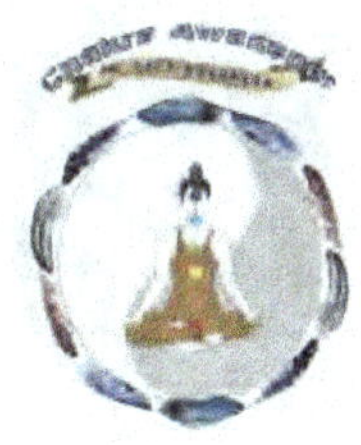

Green crystal energy is used to resolve blockages and to re-balance the Heart Chakra, helping us understand our own needs and emotions clearly. We can deal with the ebbs and flows of emotional relationships, understand their cyclic nature, and accept the changes.

Bloodstone Spiritual Energy

Bloodstone is a stone of courage and wisdom, noble sacrifice and altruistic character. It stimulates the urge toward Christ consciousness within the self and helps bring one's true spirituality into everyday life in a grounded and real way. It is also a stone of mysticism, providing insights and the spiritual intuition of truths which transcend ordinary understanding.

Bloodstone grounds and protects the soul on many levels, heightening intuition, dispelling mental confusion, and keeping out negativity and undesirable entities. Because its colors can change in different lights, it is regarded as a shape-shifting stone, teaching one to travel invisibly between the worlds and negotiate different realms. One of its most important uses has been to gain admittance to the spiritual realms of the ancestors for healing the ancestral line. By dispelling negative patterns it allows one to live in the present untrammeled by the past.

I Am Whole

How to Give Yourself a Chakra Selfie

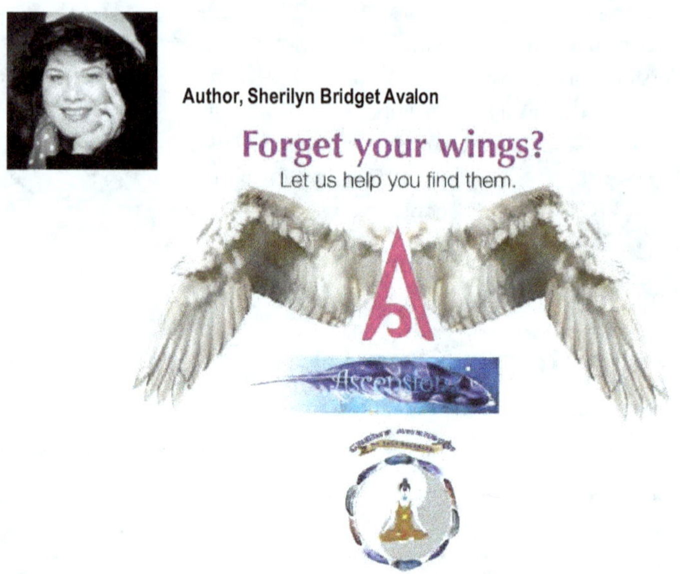

Utilize the Tesla coil violet ray and light beam applications with noble gases to balance the field and correct reverse polarity conditions, and assist in sealing the field from auric bleeding.

Tesla's Violet Ray Therapy

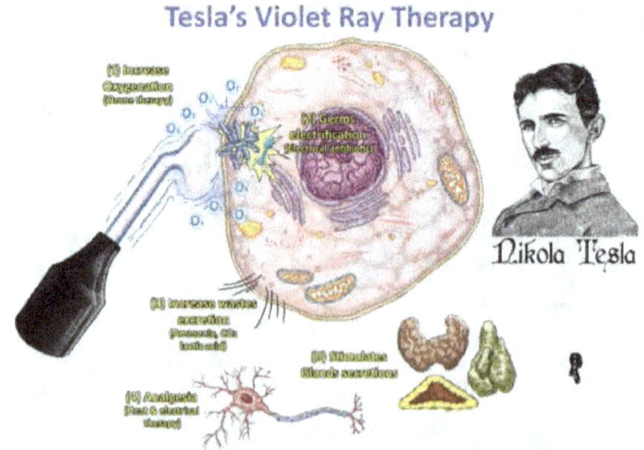

How to Give Yourself a Chakra Selfie

My last words - Our physical bodies, even our very cells, and the DNA, respond to our thoughts and our emotional focus. We must stay aware of where we direct not only our thoughts but our emotional power, as well. Are you processing and healthily releasing your emotions? Or are they building up somewhere within your physical or energetic systems? *Where do you think all that stagnant, negative energy goes when you don't release it?*

Well, a lot of negative energy gets trapped in your ethereal body. Which is the same body that looks just like your physical body, but it's pure energy.

Crystal Sound Therapy removes negative blocks.

Book an appointment at www.Ascensions.US

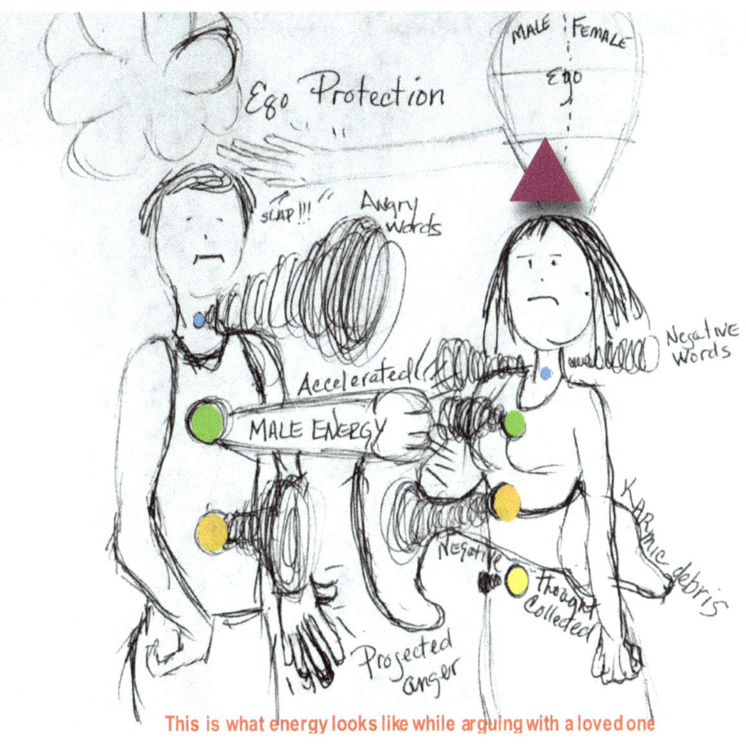

This is what energy looks like while arguing with a loved one

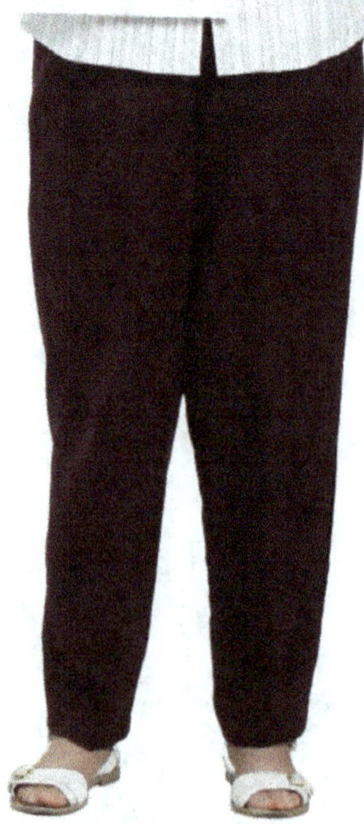
Hi, Julie here, to tell you to stay with it. Just like any new thing it takes time to form a habit. Keep practicing and it will become part of your lifestyle just like exercising, Good Luck!

Then you will feel better, be healthier.

Be aware of your Self Talk

YOUR VOICE COMMANDS YOUR MIND, BODY & SPIRIT

Learn the true meaning of each word, the root and the original intention. Find the cousins to each word, say it, feel it, which one will move you forward in your own life?

ENERGY + VIBRATION = MATTER

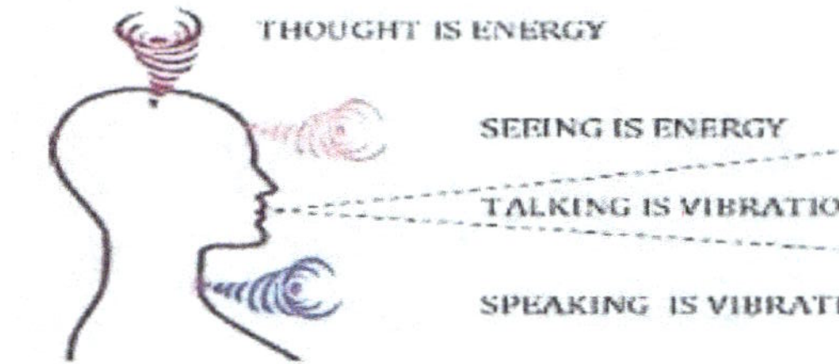

THOUGHTS + VOICE = REALITY

Help the self by Walking the Absolute Truth of your own life, Meditate & Pray...Keep thoughts, actions & words positive...Be self empowered and use the tools presented in a good way

I can't I won't It's hard I Don't Believe I'm a skeptic I don't like it	=	• Will literally stop growth • Will literally put a block in your way • Can not is a command to self • Will literally stop you from achieving anything in your life • Is a taught behavior that is a conditional to hold a person back • Stops a person from learning • Stops a person from gaining intellect (iQ)
Try Trying I can try I'm trying I will try I will attempt	=	• Try and you will do it over and over and over never get to the end • Puts a block in your way • Try is a command to self • Try and trying is a taught behavior that is a condition to hold a person back • It has very little or no results • It is like running a race with no end • It is never ending • It is repetitious
I can I am I believe It is done I can do it I can do anything	=	• Literally promotes growth • Can is a command to self • Allows your wants, needs and desire to come true • Is a behavior of using good words • It is unconditional and moves a person forward in life • When you know inside you can do it your body needs to hear it • Your body reacts to key words

49

Meditation

As you stand directly in the rays of the sun, visualize a prism floating before you. See the light of the sun, pure and white, coming down in a single direct ray.

Now visualize the ray hitting the prism. The colors instantly explode in separate waves, pulsing with life-giving energy. Each ray flows towards you.

Watch as they reach your individual chakras. As the waves of color touch your chakras, feel the warmth, fill the wheel center, expanding out through your whole body.

We all know of the sun's life-giving properties. Through stepping outside every day and visualizing the frequency of its rays, balancing our chakra system, we can reap the fullest benefits of the power of its energy body.

No chakra shall be missed for balancing: the Root, the sacral, the solar plexus, the heart, the throat, the third eye, and the crown. Each feels the heat of the ray beaming through the prism.

Sit for a few moments longer, feeling the warmth, envisioning the all-encompassing light opening your chakra centers outside of your body, and bringing harmony to your entire being mind, body, and spirit.

Your job on Earth is not to learn, but to remember **Who You Are.**
It is your sole purpose. That is, your Soul Purpose.

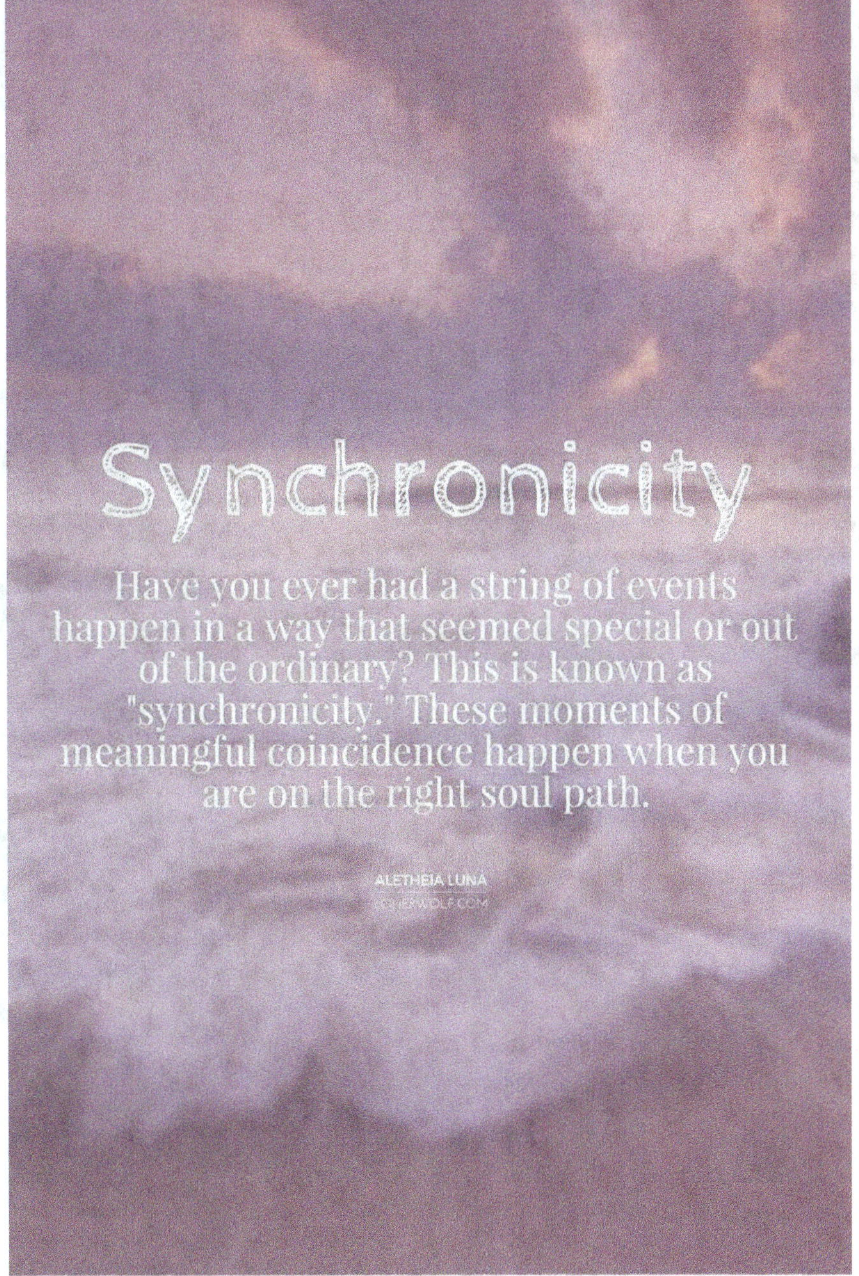
Synchronicity
Have you ever had a string of events happen in a way that seemed special or out of the ordinary? This is known as "synchronicity." These moments of meaningful coincidence happen when you are on the right soul path.
ALETHEIA LUNA
LONERWOLF.COM

Chakra Name	Chakra Symbols	Aromatherapy	Crystal Therapy
Crown ~ Sahasrara		Rosewood	Amethyst Lepidolite Clear Quartz
Third Eye ~ Anja		Cajeput Lemongrass Violet	Lapis Lazuli iolite Moldavite
Throat ~ Vishuddha		Camphor Eucalyptus Peppermint	Sodalite Blue Lace Agate Turquoise
Heart ~ Anahata		Rose Jasmine Tarragon	Rose Quartz Moss agate Emerald
Solar Plexus ~ Manipura		Lavender Chamomile Lemon	Citrine Amber Tiger's Eye
Sacral ~ Svadhishthana		Orange Myrrh Sandalwood	Goldstone Carnelian Coral
Root ~ Muladhara		Clove Rosemary Cypress	Ruby Garnet Hematite

Yoga	Color Therapy	Herbal Therapy
Headstand Rabbit	Purple White	Lavender flowers and lotus
Eye Asanas	indigo	St. John's Wort Spruce Eyebright
Fish Camel Shoulder stand	Blue	Peppermint Sage Coltsfoot
Cobra Fish Camel	Green	White Horn Thyme Melissa
Table Boat Camel	Yellow	Fennel Chamomile Juniper
Down Dog Cat Cow Fish	Orange	Nettle Yarrow Parsley
Bridge Head to Knee Knee to Chest	Red	Valerian Lime Blossom Elder Dandelion

Crystal Power

Crystal energy used on chakras

Clear Quartz: The Master Healer

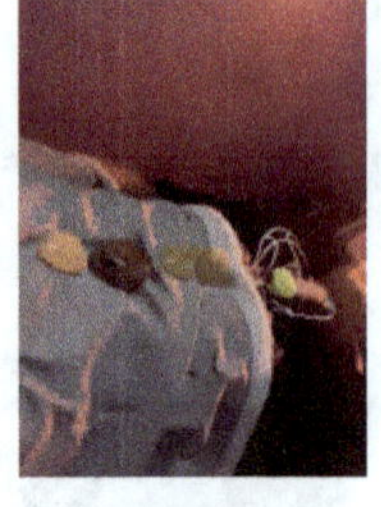

An essential crystal healing tool and the right choice for your first crystal. Do not be fooled into thinking this crystal is dull. Clear Quartz crystals are probably the most versatile crystals and can be **programmed** for any purpose.

Amethyst: The Psychic Powerhouse

It may be suitable for beginners, but it can still blow your socks off. Super spiritual Amethyst connects you with your spiritual power. Deeply cleansing, this violet crystal purifies negative energies. You can also use Amethyst for protection and developing your natural psychic abilities.

Tiger's Eye: The Confidence Builder

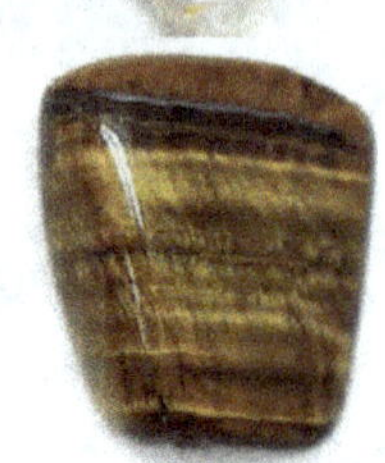

This banded golden-brown stone carries a more masculine energy. An ideal crystal for helping build confidence and self-belief. You can also use Tiger's Eye for protection. This golden stone connects us with the Earth, making it an excellent choice for grounding yourself.

Rose Quartz: The Earth Mother

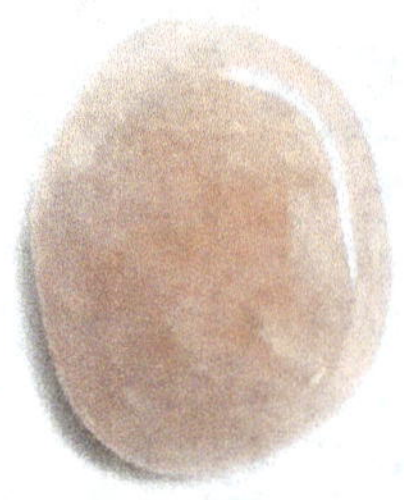

Possibly the ultimate comfort crystal. Rose Quartz is the mother of all crystals. Gentle and soothing, Rose Quartz helps heal emotional pain. Opening the Heart Chakra, it allows you to feel compassion for others and yourself. This is the self-love stone.

Why is it Important for me to learn about my Chakras?

A. Every emotion has its own vibrational frequency which affect your Chakras to help you achieve whole body wellness.

The following information is for you to do a self-analysis to increase the energy centers (Chakra's) you rated lowest.

Understanding what <u>thoughts or issues</u> may cause a chakra to stagnate (not develop fully) is key in gaining more self-knowledge.

The statements on next page are to help you with your self-analysis. These questions are for you to reflect on, and if you feel that you may be having problems in certain areas, then try bringing in color through different methods, adding crystals or colored clothing.

Chakra tools can be found on my site www.Ascensions.us

Or other sites that sell metaphysical tools.

Color speaks to the spiritual quality of matter. Most people see virtually in black and white. Those who don't are at the opposite end of the color spectrum. They see colors other people don't see. Violet is particularly important. Blue is of great consequence.

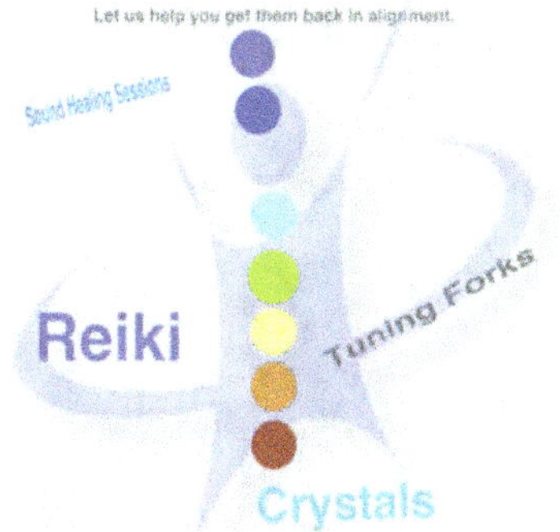

How to Give Yourself a Chakra Selfie

Most IMPORTANT

Your Root Chakra's (red power) is your connection to grounding. The Root Chakra is your central power station, and it is connected to your physical vitality and endurance, mental perseverance. It is the center that gives you your life's passion. The Root center is also your connection to your existence.

You must bring in a New Spiritual Vision. You can Affirm: " I AM thankful that God/Source perfectly provides for me all my physical needs. I gratefully accept!"

Issues to review are:

- Are you physically fit? **Rate 1-10**

- Was there or is there currently any abuse

  (physical or verbal) in your life? **Rate 1-10**

- Are you able to put your thoughts into action?
  Rate 1-10

- Do you accomplish most of your goals? **Rate 1-10**

- Are money and home very important to you?
  Rate 1-10

- Have you had any recent thoughts of self-destruction?
  Rate 1-10

How to Give Yourself a Chakra Selfie

Let's work with Crystals and I am Affirmations- I am Love

Affirmations are positive statements that have the function of strengthening and healing damaged parts of ourselves. When working with affirmations, we can focus on various aspects of ourselves to repair them. We enhance affirmations by adding Crystals. Here are some examples of affirmations for the various Chakras and their Crystals: **Take a deep breath before each affirmation.**

- **The Root Chakra -** "I am filled with humility. I am enough as I am." Garnet & Ruby.

- **The Sacral Chakra-** "I am radiant, beautiful, and strong and enjoy a healthy and passionate life." Carnelian & Coral

- **The Solar Plexus -** "I accept myself completely. I accept that I have strengths, and I accept that I have weaknesses."
Citrine & Amber.

- **The Heart Chakra -** "Love is the answer to everything in life, and I give and receive love unconditionally."
Rose Quartz & Malachite.

- **The Throat Chakra -** "My thoughts are positive, and I always express myself truthfully and clearly." Sodalite & Turquoise.

- **The Third Eye Chakra -** "I am wise, and I understand the true meaning of life's situations." Lapis Lazuli & Iolite.

- **The Crown Chakra -** "I am complete and one with the divine Chakra Alignment Services. Amethyst & Lepidolite.

https://youtu.be/b7JS0O3pFS8 Play this while doing your chakra tune-up.

Let's work with Mantras and Mudras

The Sanskrit word *mantra-* is derived from the root word **man- "to think** the suffix *-tra* designates a "tool" or instrument." Hence, a literal translation would be "a tool for thinking" or "an instrument of thought.

My thoughts are we are all Gods Thoughts.

Because it says in the Bible, in the beginning, God created Man.

Q. When using the hand (Mudras), does it open your chakras?

A. Yes! Mudras do open your chakras. These are a few.

Prana Life -Make a peace sign but keep the index & middle fingers together. (Handful of flowers) Hands in lap, palms up, thumbs gently touching.

Solar Plexus - Hakini -Fingertips together pointing away from the body, cross thumbs gently.

Gyan- Make the OK sign with the left-hand. Keep the sign at the base of the sternum; keep the right hand resting on the knee.

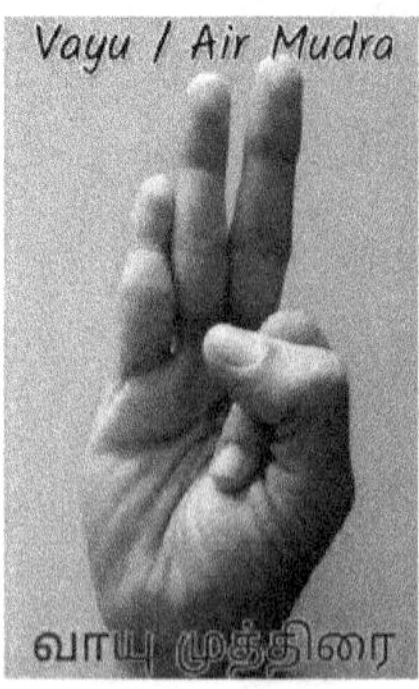

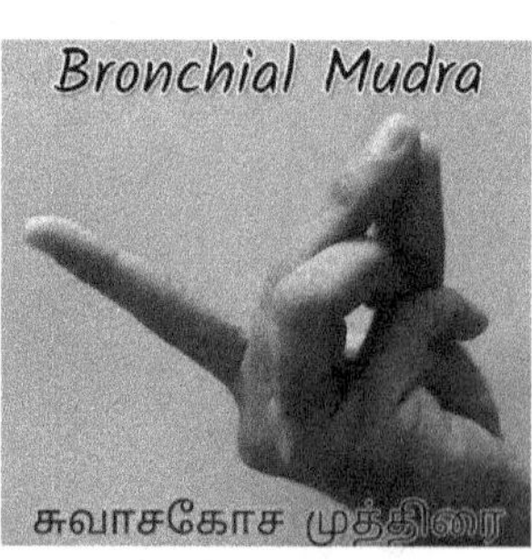

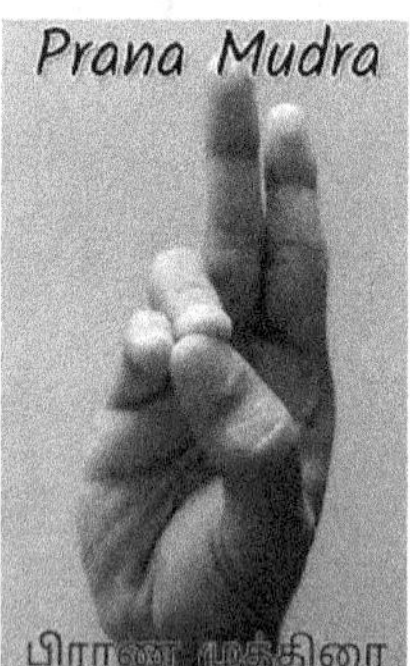

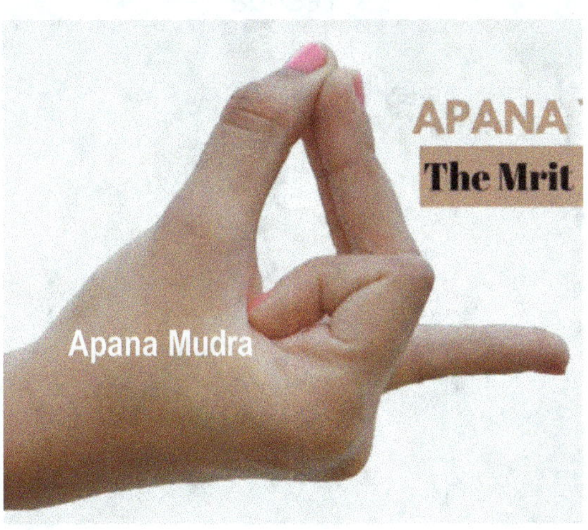

Apana Mudra

Instructions: Connect the tip of your thumb to the tips of the middle and ring fingers while keeping the other fingers extended. Allow the backs of the hands to rest on your knees or thighs.

Benefits:

Apana Vayu (Vayu is Sanskrit for "wind") is a downward moving current of energy, which helps with elimination and therefore with detoxification of the body. It can also help with digestion, both mental and physical, that are believed to occur at the solar plexus, the area above the navel. You might try this mudra if you're constipated or when you feel like you're holding onto something physically, mentally, or emotionally that you're ready to let go of.

Yeshua

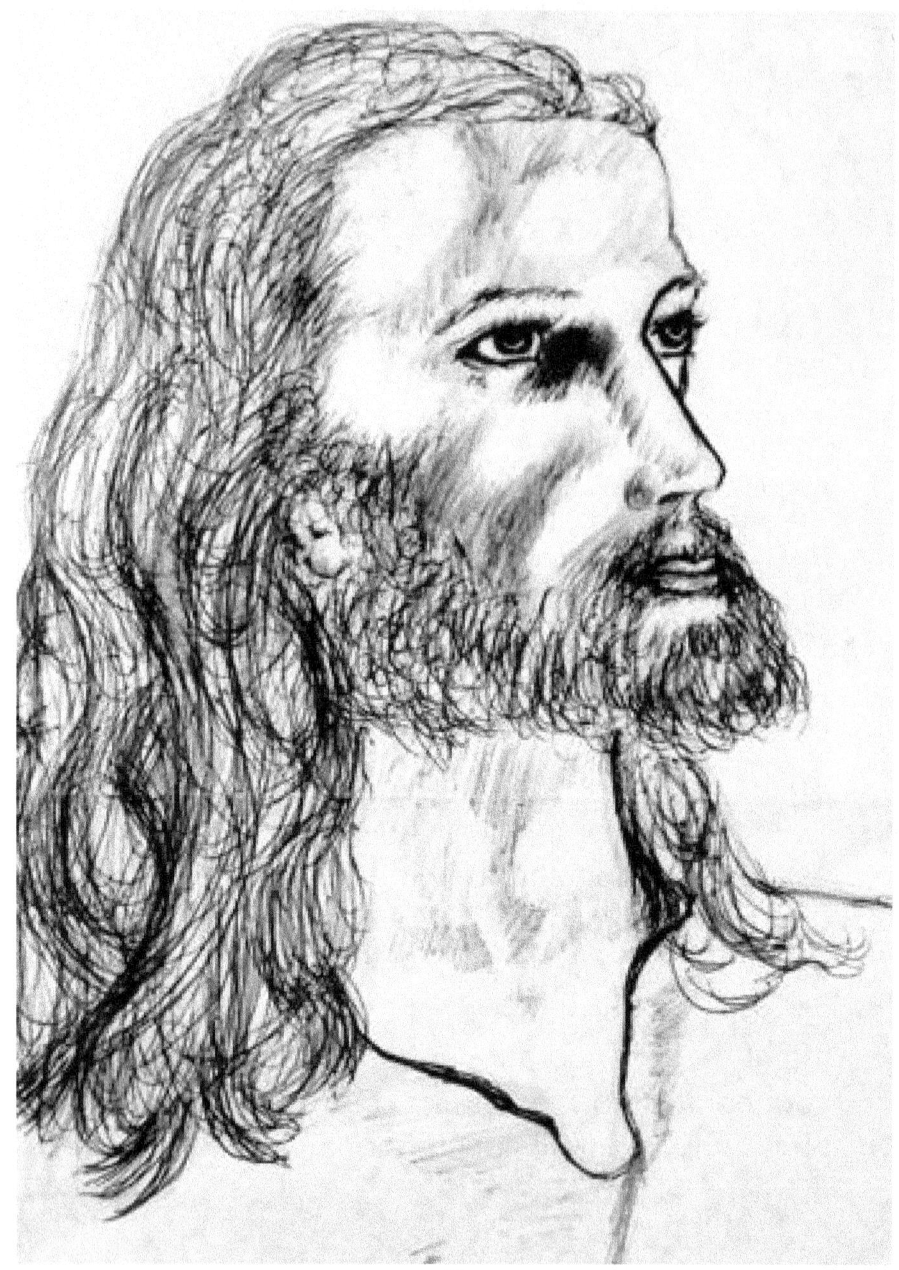

Yeshua

An optimal aura can have at its beckoning an inexhaustible force of energy. That energy is a projection from the Divine Self, the Integral Self that you can and will, in time, learn to express physically. The energy held in storage in 'Mer-Ka-Na' Crysto-lite body, is first passed into an intact Auric Field. When it carries such refined energy, it is the very essence of creatorship. It is the magic stardust of Merlin's wand. It is the esoteric fuel, the gas in the 'creation' tank. So, know that the tank must not have leaks in order to take you very far in the physical reality in which you dwell.

Archangel Metatron via Tyberonn Channel

To better understand our chakras, a.k.a. energy centers that govern different aspects of our body and mind. Our Chakras develop over our lifespan and can be related back to our physical, emotional, and spiritual health. Awareness of each chakra can help us address old wounds and balance certain aspects of our lives. Issues such as scarcity mindset, lack of confidence, difficulty with expression, or trouble making decisions can be improved with this knowledge. Our experiences and our ability to process emotions can affect our chakras development and when any one of them are imbalanced it will eventually affect all of them. When you bring your chakras to their original vibration, you can create more harmony within yourself and the world around you.

Connect with your breath exercise

You can't master that which you don't understand. We are empowered by understanding our **Chakra** system. For within this system lies the most important aspect of who we are as **humans, spiritual music, intention, and the healing power from the human voice, also energetic treatments can be produced specific to each person's needs.** Within the treatment a variety of frequencies can be combined that might include **frequencies** through colored light energetics or Chakra Selfie healings that will encourage and improve the body's natural healing abilities.

Training Journal info

Lay down with your Chakra Selfie Stick ™ You can choose your left hand or your right hand to hold it, imagine you are going to trace a circle around your Chakras.

Start at the bottom, your root Chakra, pause, and continue tracing your Chakra's energy, pause, watch your pendulum move back and forth, or in circular motion notice how it feels. Keep going until you have finished tracing all your Chakra's to your seventh Chakra (Crown).

Now you are ready to add some breathing. Breathe in through your nose and breathe out through your mouth. Remember to keep it slow and steady.

Place your Chakra Selfie Pendulum over a Chakra, it will automatically go to the one that most needed healing, and breathe in as you trace the Chakra, wheel or vortex. Breathe out as you trace the Chakra wheel. Breathe in as you slide up to your second Chakra, and breathe out as you trace second Chakra, Keep going until you have finished tracing your whole-body Chakra system, and you have taken five slow breaths, then five quick breaths. Repeat 2 or 3 times. How does your body feel now? Do you feel calm, or would you like to do another session?

THE
BREATH

TRAINING JOURNAL

BEFORE YOU BEGIN. WATCH THIS:

www.Ascensions.us/ The Breath

STARTING DATE: ___ /___ /___

PROTOCOL:

___ sets of ___ reps per session, ___ sessions per day ___ days per week with effort maintained **IN THE ZONE.**

WEEK 1	SUN		MON		TUE		WED		THU		FRI		SAT	
	AM	PM	AM	PM	AM	PM	AM	PM	AM	PM	AM	PM	AM	PM
I INHALE/EXHALE REPS/SETS COMPLETED	8													
Rate Your Effort	3													
Rotation of energy	3													

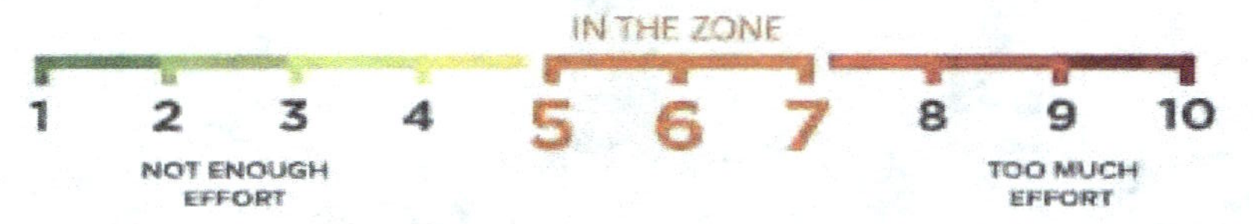

IN THE ZONE

1 2 3 4 5 6 7 8 9 10

NOT ENOUGH EFFORT

TOO MUCH EFFORT

What is breath of L.I.F.E. Breathing?
During breath of **LIFE** breathing, we concentrate on taking five slow breaths in through the nose and out through the mouth. If you notice that your breathing through the nose is a challenge, imagine you are smelling a beautiful flower or your favorite food as you breathe in, and then to breathe out with a big sigh. At the same time as breathing, focus on the action of placing the Chakra Selfie Stick over the chakras feel the gentle sensations this creates.

TRAINING

JOURNAL

STARTING DATE: _/_/_

**Inhale through the heart
Exhale through the
third eye**

WEEK 1	SUN		MON		TUE		WED		THU		FRI		SAT	
	AM	PM	AM	PM	AM	PM	AM	PM	AM	PM	AM	PM	AM	PM
INHALE/EXHALE														
REPS/SETS COMPLETED														
Rotation of Energy														

WEEK 2	SUN		MON		TUE		WED		THU		FRI		SAT	
	AM	PM	AM	PM	AM	PM	AM	PM	AM	PM	AM	PM	AM	PM
INHALE/EXHALE														
REPS/SETS COMPLETED														
Rotation of Energy														

WEEK 3	SUN		MON		TUE		WED		THU		FRI		SAT	
	AM	PM	AM	PM	AM	PM	AM	PM	AM	PM	AM	PM	AM	PM
INHALE/EXHALE														
REPS/SETS COMPLETED														
Rotation of Energy														

WEEK 4	SUN		MON		TUE		WED		THU		FRI		SAT	
	AM	PM	AM	PM	AM	PM	AM	PM	AM	PM	AM	PM	AM	PM
INHALE/EXHALE														
REPS/SETS COMPLETED														
Rotation of Energy														

What is breath of L.I.F.E. Breathing?
During breath of **LIFE** breathing, we concentrate on taking five slow breaths in through the nose and out through the mouth. If you notice that your breathing through the nose is a challenge, imagine you are smelling a beautiful flower or your favorite food as you breathe in, and then to breathe out with a big sigh. At the same time as breathing, focus on the action of placing the Chakra Selfie Stick over the chakras feel the gentle sensations this creates.

TRAINING

JOURNAL

STARTING **DATE:** _/_/_

Inhale through the heart
Exhale through the
third eye

WEEK 1	SUN		MON		TUE		WED		THU		FRI		SAT	
	AM	PM	AM	PM	AM	PM	AM	PM	AM	PM	AM	PM	AM	PM
INHALE/EXHALE														
REPS/SETS COMPLETED														
Rotation of Energy														

WEEK 2	SUN		MON		TUE		WED		THU		FRI		SAT	
	AM	PM	AM	PM	AM	PM	AM	PM	AM	PM	AM	PM	AM	PM
INHALE/EXHALE														
REPS/SETS COMPLETED														
Rotation of Energy														

WEEK 3	SUN		MON		TUE		WED		THU		FRI		SAT	
	AM	PM	AM	PM	AM	PM	AM	PM	AM	PM	AM	PM	AM	PM
INHALE/EXHALE														
REPS/SETS COMPLETED														
Rotation of Energy														

WEEK 4	SUN		MON		TUE		WED		THU		FRI		SAT	
	AM	PM	AM	PM	AM	PM	AM	PM	AM	PM	AM	PM	AM	PM
INHALE/EXHALE														
REPS/SETS COMPLETED														
Rotation of Energy														

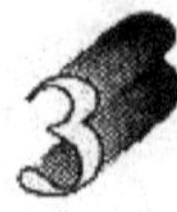

3 steps to the fulfillment of your dreams
STEP 1
Self Hypnosis and Beyond

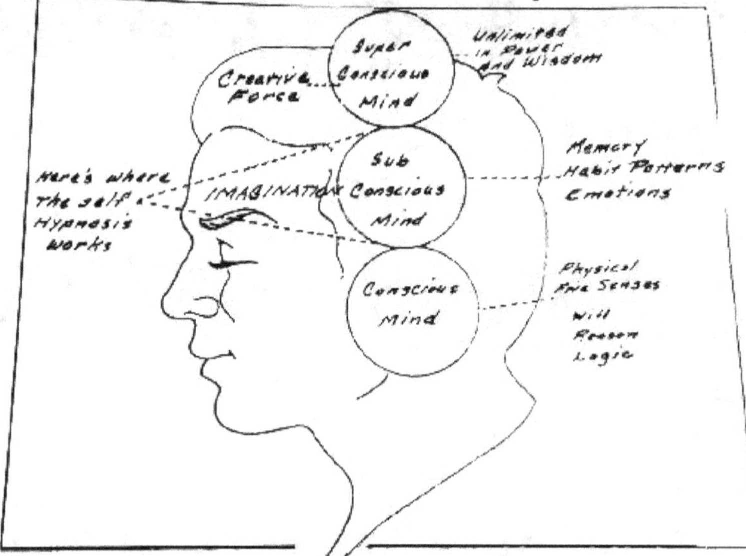

The Key To Inner Self Discovery

What I Learned with Don Weldon I made this for him.

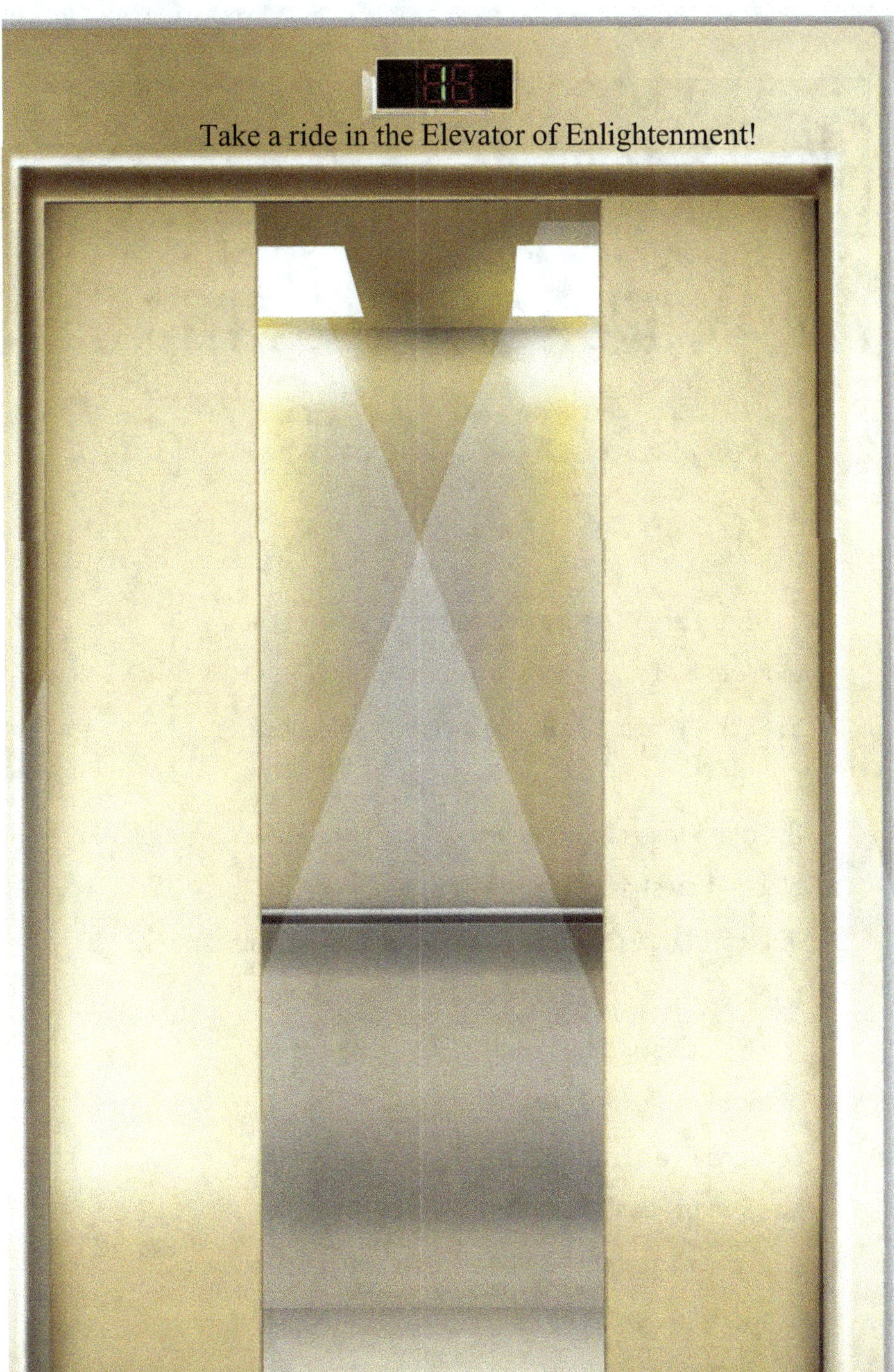
Take a ride in the Elevator of Enlightenment!

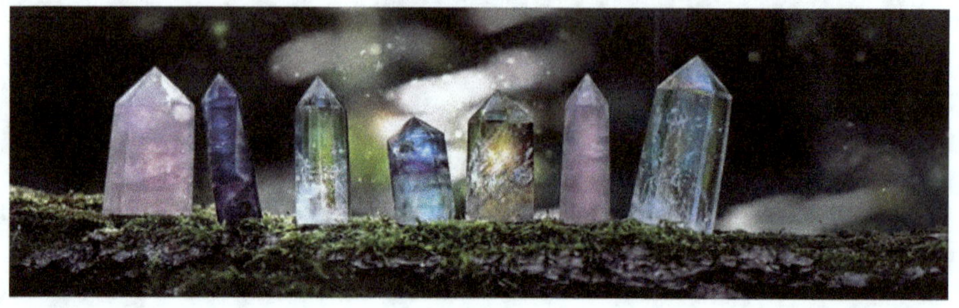

Crystals, do they really work?

1. Root **Earth Chakra** - Deals with survival. It's blocked by fear.

2. Sacral **Water Chakra** - Deals with pleasure. It's blocked by guilt.

3. Solar Plexus **Fire Chakra** - Deals with power. It's blocked by shame.

4. Heart **Love Chakra** - Deals with love. It's blocked by grief.

5. Throat **Sound Chakra** - Deals with truth. It's blocked by lies that we tell ourselves.

6. Third Eye **Light Chakra**- Deals with insight. It's blocked by illusion.

7. Crown **Thought Chakra** - Deals with pure cosmic energy. it's blocked by all earthling attachment.

Crystal Singing Bowls

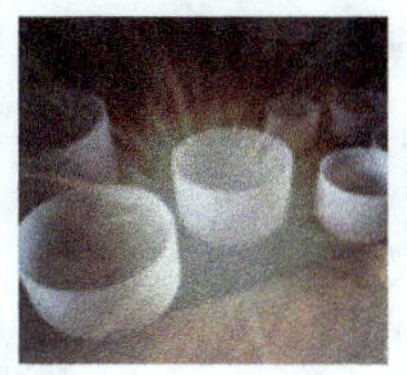

WHAT ARE CRYSTAL SINGING BOWLS?

Singing Bowls produce a harmonization between their vibration and that of the person. Resonance is the principle on which vibrational medicine works. Resonance is the capacity of a certain vibration to produce a response in something with a similar vibration. The vibration of Crystal bowls has the power to make atoms vibrate and reorganize themselves in a crystalline structure, which is stronger, healthier and more balanced. The sound will affect the whole individual in a holistic manner, balancing first the energetic body and chakras and then cleaning the auric field. The vibration spikes the spinal cord which acts as a strong resonance vehicle sending the waves through the nervous system, cells, tissue and organs. These tones or vibrations bring the individual playing or listening into heightened states of consciousness because of the effect on inter-neuronal connections. The sound waves produced by the bowls induce a state of relaxation similar to the practice of long-term meditation. While in this relaxed state induced by the bowls the mind guides the consciousness on an inner journey giving sensation of what Zen Masters call "filling oneself up with emptiness". This state of emptiness gives us the opportunity to see the world and ourselves from a different perspective.

HOW WILL SINGING BOWLS MAKE ME FEEL?

The people who experience the effects of the bowls describe it as a deep physical and mental relaxation, sensations of floating and wellbeing. The experience can unblock and dissolve energetic and physical obstructions in the physical and astral body and thus is a therapeutic tool for deep healing. This is because the seven musical notes reverberate in the 7 chakras, and the 7 colors of the human aura creating a vibrational bath which emits a natural balancing effect.

SCIENCE BEHIND THE BOWLS

Modern quantum theory tells us that everything is essentially energy. When two quanta of similar vibration are united matter is formed, meaning all matter is composed of a different frequency of particles in movement. So too, all organic forms are created by the quantum field with similar vibrations, our bodies, organs, muscles, tissue etc. If bacteria or any other organism with a different vibration enters our bodies, it alters the vibrational model, producing illness. This is where sound therapy gives the best results as it can realign the affected tissue. Resonance is the principle on which vibrational medicine works.

How do I clean my crystals?
There are several methods to energetically clean your crystals.

Cleansing Methods for All

Crystals

Is my crystal okay in Salt?

Only Crystals that have a hardness of at least 3 on the Mohs Scale

Smoke -

Just like smoke clears out your home or office space energetically, it is great for clearing out your crystals.

Singing Bowls -
Negative energy buildup and replace it with positive. This can be done in a metal Tibetan singing bowl or a Quartz crystal bowl. You could also take the crystals to a sound bath with you.

Tuning Forks -
You could also gently place the end of the fork directly on the stone.

→ **Returning to the earth.** Burying your crystals in the earth is another favorite. It grounds the energy back to Source and allows your stone to take a little nap. You can bury your crystals in a potted plant, in your garden, or in the sand at the beach.

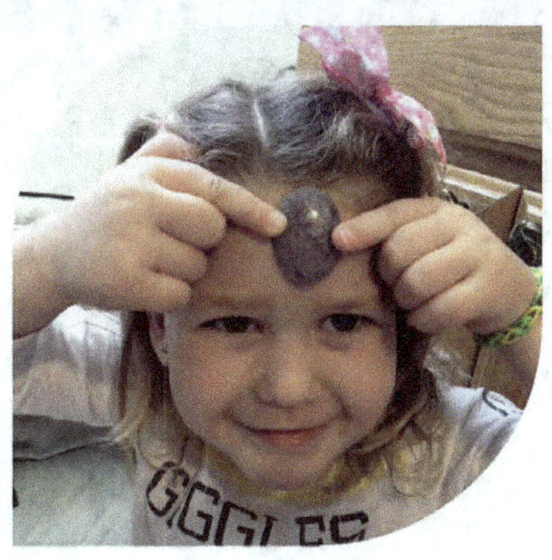

2.5. To be on the safe side, we recommend your stones to be on Mohs Scale of Hardness, you will be able to scratch anything below at least a 3.

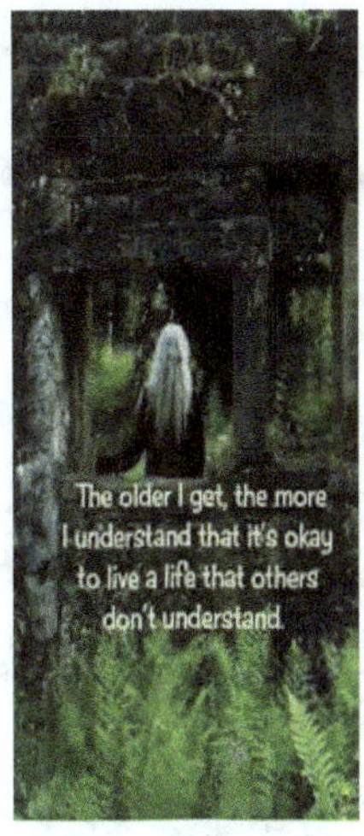

Mohs Hardness Scale

Mineral Name	Scale Number	Common Object
Diamond	10	
Corundum	9	
Masonry Drill Bit	8	
Topaz	8/4	
Quartz	7	
Orthoclase	6	
Steel Nail	6.5	
Knife/Glass Plate	5.5	
Apatite	5	
Calcite	2.5	
Gypsum	2	

How will Holding a Crystal Pyramid make me Feel?

Holding a pyramid is a joyful experience, and the more you practice, the more joy you generate.

Top 7 Crystal Pyramid Uses.

Here are the top seven ways you can make use of your crystal pyramid. Below the list, we expand on each method.

1. Crystal pyramid energy healing for the aura and 7 chakras.

2. Crystal pyramid meditations for clairvoyance and high spiritual vibration.

3. Program crystal pyramids with reiki intentions for love, healing, money etc.

4. Focus upon a crystal pyramid while you do yoga.

5. Place the crystal pyramid in your room to preserve youth and beauty.

6. Make pyramid elixirs to drink for good health and physical preservation

7. Place the pyramid in your fridge to energize and preserve food.

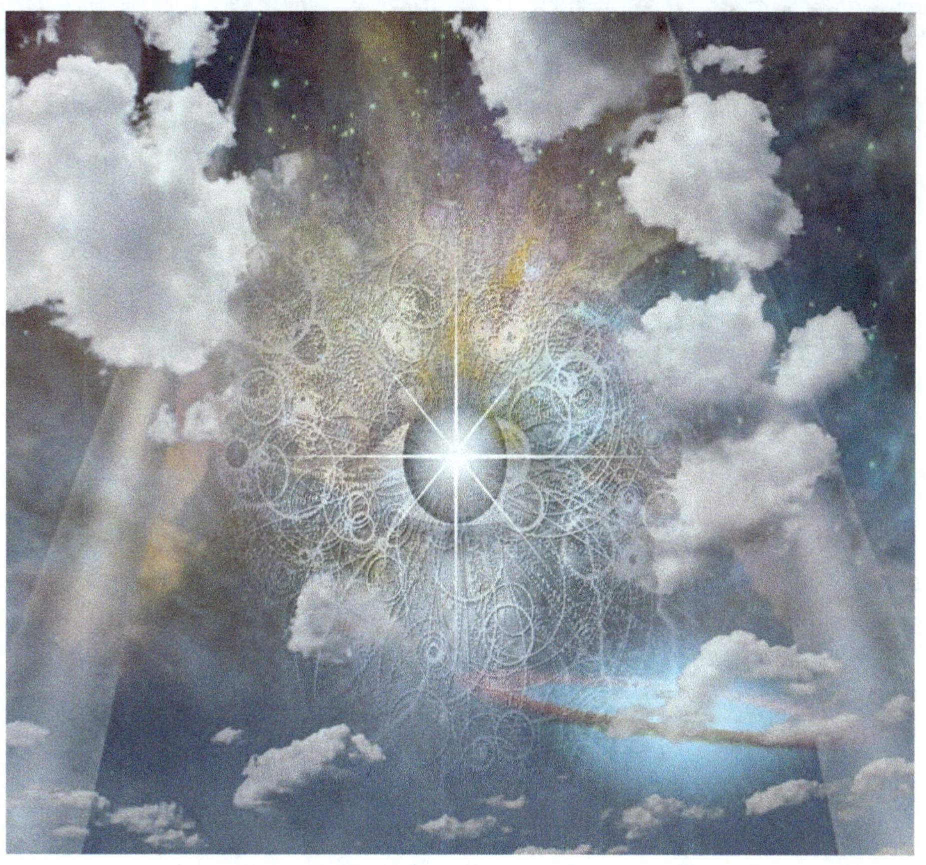

Q. How do I Use a Crystal Pyramid during Meditation?

To use a Crystal Pyramid for Meditation, place it directly in your hand or in front of you while you engage in your session. If you have a meditation space, it can be placed anywhere within that room or sacred area. The pyramid naturally vibrates at the spiritual level because it is an important form of sacred geometry. The energy of the pyramid helps to raise vibrations so you can achieve the next level of spiritual development.

The Top 7 Crystal Pyramid Uses Explained

Q1. How Do I Use Crystal Pyramids for Energy Healing?

Surround yourself with pyramids. To benefit quickly and intensively from Pyramid Power, you can form a grid of pyramids around your body as you do a crystal layout or even while you sleep. The pyramids will draw down energy effortlessly, and your body vibrations will increase.

Q2. How do I use a Crystal Pyramid to Preserve Food?

Maximize the preservation powers of the crystal pyramid by placing it in your fridge to preserve food. Doing so not only increases the shelf life of your food, but also keeps the nutritional values intact.

Q3. How do I Program my Crystal Pyramids for Reiki?

Pyramids are perfect for Reiki, because Reiki operates on important universal symbols. Infuse Reiki energy into your pyramid to intensify powers. When you input your intentions into a crystal it helps focus the healing benefits to your needs. This can be for more love, money, health, spirituality, or anything you desire.

Q4. How do I use Crystal Pyramids while doing Yoga?

To benefit from crystal pyramid power while doing yoga, keep a crystal pyramid within your range of site to get more energized.

Q5. How do I use Crystal Pyramids while sleeping? *To use the crystal pyramid for preserving beauty and youth, place it near your bedside. The pyramid will bring restful sleep, which in turn preserves your appearance. Another pyramid should be placed near your mirror or vanity, the place where your self-care.*

Q6. How do I make a crystal pyramid elixir for good health?

Place your crystal pyramid in or next to your water jug to make an elixir. Keep the stone there for 1-2 hours. This will energize your water supply and convert into a direct physical benefit once you drink it. The pyramid power will help you preserve good health and your physical body.

Please note that the pyramid must be cleaned before placing in the elixir. Also, not all stones can be used to make elixirs, as some may cause negative effects. Selenite and Angelite, for example, cannot be in water because they are soft stones that will eventually dissolve.

Two types of Crystal Pyramids.

1. the one I'm holding which is Tubular. 2. A solid Crystal Pyramid.

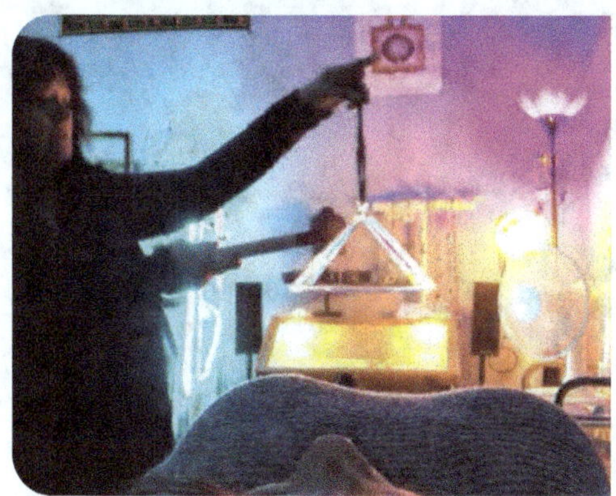

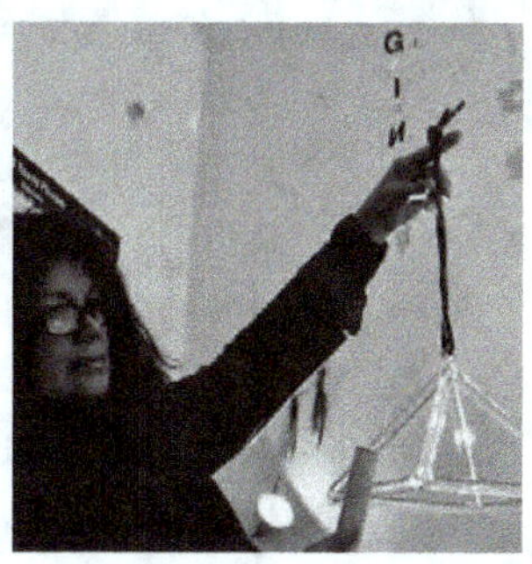

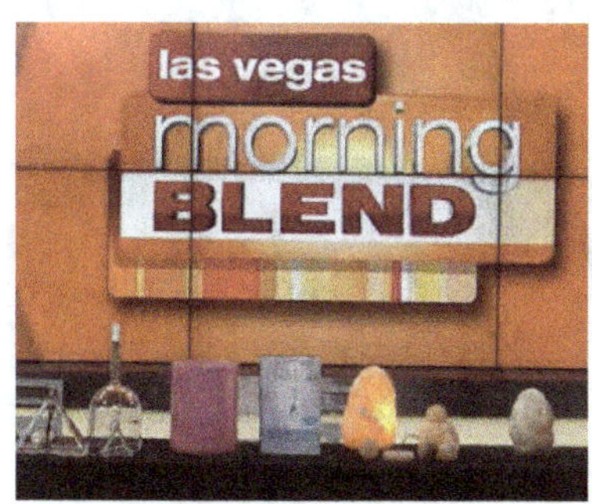

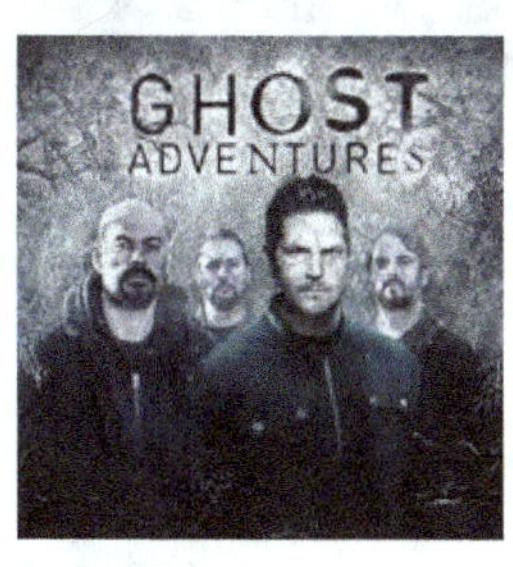

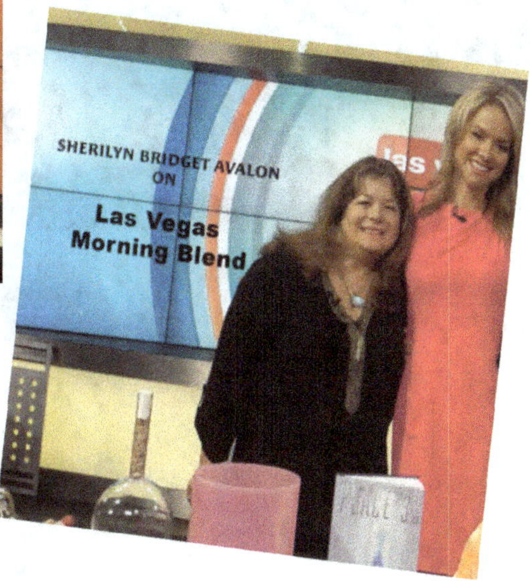

Sherilyn B. Avalon

As seen on Las Vegas Morning Blend and Ghost Adventures.

Be Informed of Blocked Chakras

How do you know when your Root chakra is blocked?

When your Root chakra is blocked, you have very little will to live. Depending on the severity of the block, you could feel a little lethargic all the way to suicidal.

This chakra imbalance can lead to restlessness, anger, rage, low self-esteem, pessimism, narrow mindedness, anxiety, overthinking, and nightmares. Because you are not properly rooted to the earth, you could show signs of greed, waste and destruction of nature. www.Ascensions.us

We can begin to see the perspective that changes everything when we... **Step 1.** *View everyone in your life as a messenger that is here to show you your inner world.* **Step 2.** *When you feel triggered by a person or experience, mentally remove the messenger and ask yourself, "Where in my body do I feel this emotion/energetic charge.* **Step 3.** *Once you identify where in the body this is felt, give yourself full permission to fully feel it without trying to change or manipulate it in any way.* **Step 4.** *Once it is felt allow the energy to move and release/integrate into your being naturally. This practice has set me free from a constant state of reaction and propelled me into a grounded, present place of response.*

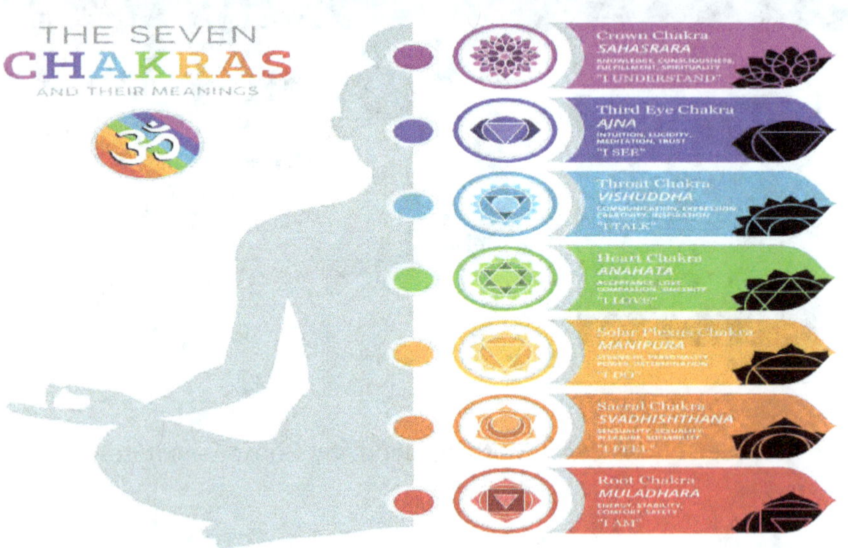

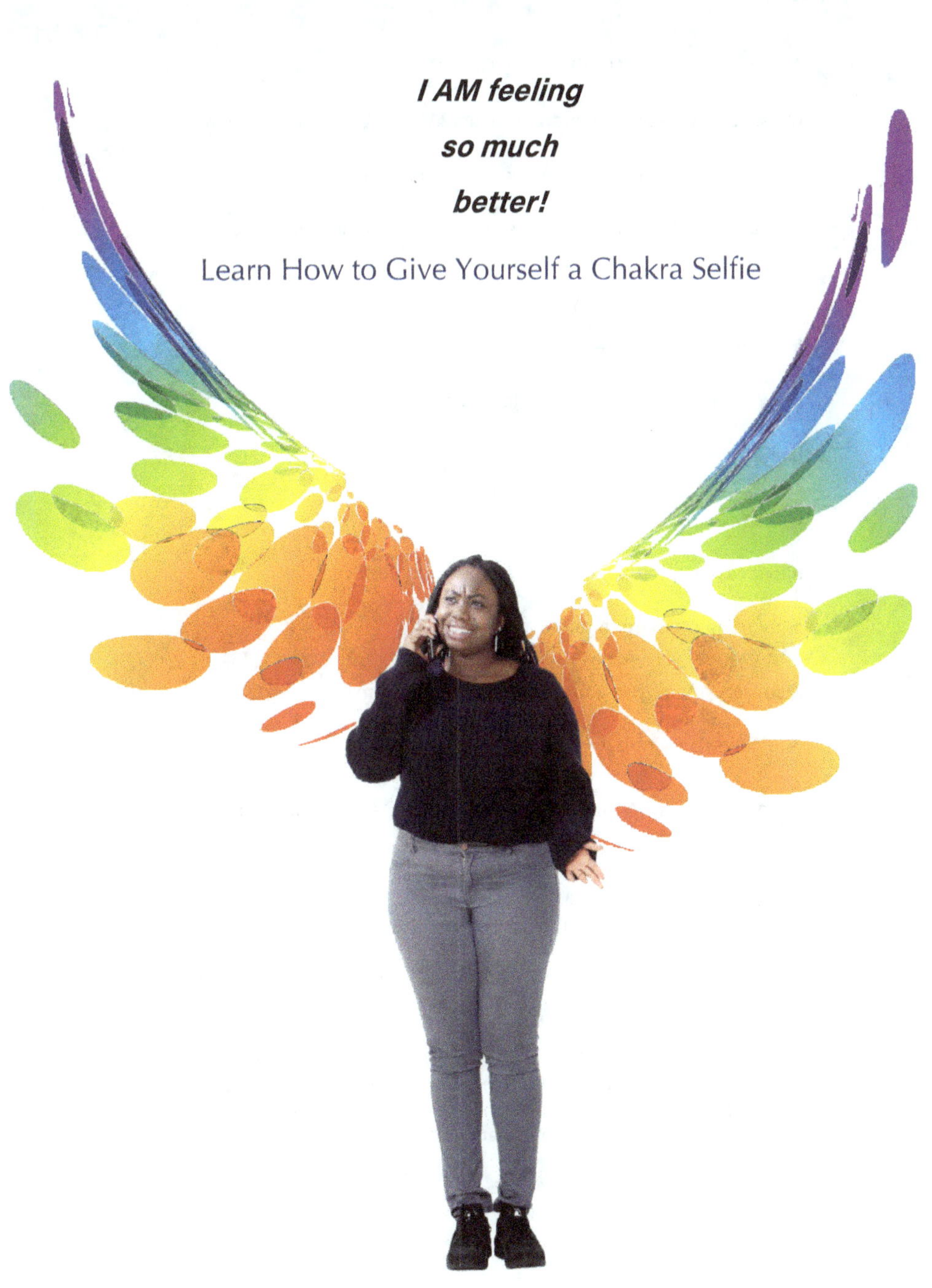

I AM feeling

so much

better!

Learn How to Give Yourself a Chakra Selfie

Resources

The Human Aura | IN SERVICE TO SPIRIT.

https://inservicetospirit.wordpress.com/2017/05/26/the-human-aura/

S h i e l d i n g Yourself From Negative Energies -

spiritualunite.com. https://www.spiritualunite.com/articles/shielding-

yourself-

from-negative-energies/

www.indianinthemachine.wordpress.com/category/transforming-to-

higher-self/page/14/

Under-active Crown

https://www.spiritualunite.com/articles/underactive-

crown-chakra-symptoms/"

Mudras - https://www.brettlarkin.com/apana-mudra/

The Seven Rainbow Flames

Affirmations from Adama -From The Seven Sacred Flames by Aurelia.

The Crysto-Electric Auric Manifold Effect & Auric Effects of Air Travel

JANUARY 24, 2012ADMIN

AA Metatron via James Tyberonn | January 24, 2012

MASTERS, as humans in duality you have become so filtered from your true identity that you no longer recognize your creatorship. Truly you are immortal beings of the Divine. You are nonphysical. That you term the auric field is much closer to your actual essence than the biological clothing you temporarily wear.